"Now, this is a consumer guide worth owning! Drs. Giannetti and Booms have written the ultimate guide for anyone needing a clear, concise understanding of the orthodontic process. *Beyond Braces: A Consumer's Guide to Orthodontics* is the first book I've seen that addresses the very core of the patient experience by offering crisp, succinct advice on how to achieve the best results in corrective dentistry."

LADONNA DRURY-KLEIN, RDA, BS

founder and chief operations officer, The Foundation for Allied Dental Education

BEYOND
BRACES

BEYOND BRACES

A CONSUMER'S GUIDE TO ORTHODONTICS

DR. KELLY GIANNETTI • DR. THAIS BOOMS

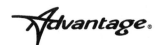

Published by Advantage, Charleston, South Carolina.
Member of Advantage Media Group.

ADVANTAGE is a registered trademark, and the Advantage colophon is a trademark of Advantage Media Group, Inc.

Printed in the United States of America.

10 9 8 7 6 5 4 3 2 1

ISBN: 978-1-64225-042-8
LCCN: 2019931996

Cover and layout design by George Stevens.

This publication is designed to provide accurate and authoritative information in regard to the subject matter covered. It is sold with the understanding that the publisher is not engaged in rendering legal, accounting, or other professional services. If legal advice or other expert assistance is required, the services of a competent professional person should be sought.

 Advantage Media Group is proud to be a part of the Tree Neutral® program. Tree Neutral offsets the number of trees consumed in the production and printing of this book by taking proactive steps such as planting trees in direct proportion to the number of trees used to print books. To learn more about Tree Neutral, please visit **www.treeneutral.com**.

Advantage Media Group is a publisher of business, self-improvement, and professional development books and online learning. We help entrepreneurs, business leaders, and professionals share their Stories, Passion, and Knowledge to help others Learn & Grow. Do you have a manuscript or book idea that you would like us to consider for publishing? Please visit **advantagefamily.com** or call **1.866.775.1696**.

We dedicate this book to all our patients and their families, and to all of you who have trusted us with your care or that of your loved ones. You have provided us invaluable lessons on orthodontic treatment and human interaction. We are delighted every time one of you chooses to become a part of our practice as you are the reason we come to work striving to be better every day.

Thank you for being a part of our journey!

ACKNOWLEDGMENTS

We want to thank our staff for making the work we do enjoyable and rewarding. In particular, we would like to thank our director of operations, Amber, who has been the backbone of our practice for twenty years. Amber, we could not do it without your support and belief in the work we do. Karen Moawad, founder of Hummingbird Consultants, also deserves a mention for her guidance and help with our professional development. We are so fortunate to be able to work with you and appreciate the high standard you hold us to. Your professionalism is inspiring.

I would also like to thank Stephen, Maya, and Isabella for supporting my passion for orthodontics. And to my mentors, who have given me the tools to succeed at the work I love.

DR. GIANNETTI

I would like to thank my family—Chris, Enzo, Lia, and my mom, Ana Maria—for supporting me on my journey. And also to all my mentors for sharing their knowledge with me.

DR. BOOMS

TABLE OF CONTENTS

ABOUT THE AUTHORS

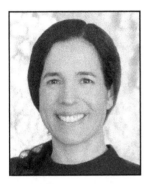

DR. THAIS BOOMS

Dr. Booms grew up in Brazil with her five siblings (four boys). Growing up, she was always fascinated with physics and biology—her father was an engineering professor and her mom a biology professor. During her training in dental school, she realized orthodontics was a combination of physics and biology and she knew then she had found what she could be forever passionate about.

While attending dental school in Brazil, Dr. Booms was always reading about orthodontics and her favorite author was a professor at the University of Michigan. Her goal became to study orthodontics at the University of Michigan and that is where she attended her three-year residency, graduating with her master's of science in orthodontics in 2001. After graduation, Dr. Booms served as an associate professor at the University of Michigan.

While in Michigan, Dr. Booms met her husband, Christopher. They relocated to Sacramento, California in 2006 in search of similar weather to Dr. Booms' hometown in Brazil (being from Michigan, Chris has been a trooper adapting to Sacramento's summers). They have two kids—Enzo and Lia—who keep them amazed and on their toes.

Dr. Booms and Chris chose Sacramento because of its outdoors opportunities—with their kids, they love camping, hiking, biking, paddle boarding and finding new swim holes in the Sierras. Dr. Booms enjoys being a part of the community where she practices and loves seeing many familiar faces at the office.

DDS, Federal University of Uberlandia, Brazil

MS in Orthodontics, University of Michigan

Diplomate, American Board of Orthodontics

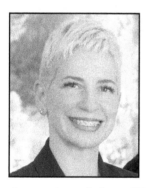

DR. KELLY GIANNETTI

Dr. Kelly Giannetti grew up in the Central Valley of California. As a child of teachers, she developed a love for education. She graduated from UC Davis with a BS in physiology and moved to Boston for her next adventure in dental school. In 1995, she graduated from Harvard University with a doctorate in dental medicine and a master's in public health. She furthered her orthodontic specialty education with a master's in oral biology at the University of California at San Francisco. After graduating in 1998, Dr. Giannetti moved to Sacramento, California to be near her family.

In addition to her private practice, Dr. Giannetti is the director of the Orthodontic Assisting Program at the FADE Institute and a guest lecturer at UCSF Orthodontic Department. Her passion for dentistry, learning, and travelling takes her to all corners of the world where she collaborates with other health care providers to bring a unique perspective to her practice.

Dr. Giannetti met her husband, Stephen, in 1986 at UC Davis. Stephen is a fine art painter whose paintings inspired the practice logo and are on display in the office. They have two girls, Maya and Isabella. Maya is currently in dental school at UCLA and hopes to join Dr. Giannetti and Dr. Booms after graduation. Isabella is a freshman in college.

BS in Physiology, University of California, Davis

DMD, and MPH, Harvard University

MS in Orthodontics, University of California, San Francisco

Diplomate, American Board of Orthodontics

Volunteer leadership positions with the California Association of Orthodontists and the Sacramento District Dental Society

Drs. Booms and Giannetti have been practicing orthodontics together since 2007. They have an invaluable combination of being trained on the East and West Coast as well as their clinical experience. Drs. Booms and Giannetti also love the perspective they have from being parents and patients themselves—their philosophy is to treat all who come to their office as they would treat their children and family. When you come to the office, you will be able to tell they are quite an incredible team who are passionate about what they do.

What to Expect at Your First Visit

by Dr. Booms

Your very first visit to an orthodontist is an important one. In most cases, the visit, exam, and consultation with the doctor will be complimentary (it is at our practice) and is your chance to meet the doctor and the team and get a feel for the office. While every practice is a little bit different, this is how booking and making your first visit to our office will proceed.

Scheduling is easy to do, and you do not need a referral from any source. It's simple to book your first appointment by going onto our website and clicking on the button marked "Make a New Patient Consultation." This allows you to look at the full appointment calendar so you can see what's available for you. If you prefer to call, we're happy to schedule that way too. Whether it's on the website or the phone, we'll ask you for some information ahead of your appointment. We'll also ask for your insurance information ahead of your visit so we can research your benefits for you before you get here.

We usually also call your dentist before you come in to confirm there are no dental barriers to orthodontic treatment that we should be aware of. That way, when you come in, we can go ahead and schedule your next appointment right away. But even if you haven't been seen by a dentist in a while, you can still come to see us, and we'll go from there. We love recommending the great dentists in your area, and we know quite a few! We want this process to be as seamless and easy for you as it can be.

On your first visit, you are going to meet our treatment coordinator, who is our new patient specialist. Her role is to walk you through all the steps and answer all the questions that you have about treatments, including what to expect during treatment, and to coordinate anything that needs to be done by different providers. If you need a dentist or a cleaning, for instance, she'll help you with that. She makes sure that everything is taken care of and that you're good to go.

Next, you'll be seen by one of our team members, who will do the necessary imaging to allow the doctor to make a proper diagnosis. Typically, these images consist of x-rays, a 3-D scan of your teeth, and photos. The doctor will then meet with you, evaluate your imaging records, and perform an examination of your face and teeth. At the end of the exam, your doctor will go over treatment options and, if treatment is recommended at that time, we will go over fees.

We love using 3-D imaging with our patients because we find that patients and parents understand the problems and the goals of treatment much more clearly when they can see images of the problems and outcome. And 3-D imaging allows us to do that: it shows them, on the screen, a simulation of their outcome! Technology is amazing!

SIX INITIAL QUESTIONS

There are six essential questions our patients often ask at this initial consultation appointment:

1. Is there an orthodontic problem, and what is it?
2. What needs to be done to correct the problem?
3. Will any teeth need to be removed?
4. Do I need headgear? Do I need an expander?
5. How long will the treatment take to complete?
6. How much will this cost?
7. Will I/my child need a retainer after treatment is done?

If there is a problem, we'll go over it with you in detail, with an emphasis on your main concerns: What brought you to our office? If you had a magic wand and could change anything about your smile/bite, what would that be? We will make sure that your concerns get addressed when we develop the treatment plan for your case.

In answering the second question, I want to stress that we design the whole treatment plan around the patient's wants and needs. So having discovered what it is that brought the patient in, we now go over the options in terms of treatment modalities—whether braces or aligners are needed, for instance—and what it will take to achieve the patient's goals. Just as every mouth is different, every treatment plan will be different too.

Just as every mouth is different, every treatment plan will be different too.

I may see other problems with a patient's teeth that they didn't notice, that also will be addressed in the treatment plan. Even so, we do our best to tailor it to the patients' needs and expectations, to make sure that we offer them a timetable that they are willing to see through, and that they know what to expect when we're done. This is important because we often see patients for second and third opinions when they have been unable to find a provider who tailored a plan to their needs, or they feel the provider did not listen to them. And we strongly believe in open communications in terms of expectations, goals, and what the patient is willing to go through.

For example, I may have a patient who, ideally, needs orthodontics plus jaw surgery. And by ideal, I mean that this combination would produce the best results in terms of the proportions of the bones, face, and bite. Orthodontists look at lots of measurements and proportions, and sometimes balancing them might require jaw surgery or tooth extraction. There are patients who are fine with those options, and there are also patients who will tell me frankly, "I'm not willing to go through all that. What are my options, and how much improvement can I get by doing something that doesn't involve surgery or having teeth removed?" I'm always willing to work with them to find a solution that yields a good long-term result while accommodating their wishes.

Delia was in that position. She was fifty-five years old and had crowded teeth and a skeletal issue: the bottom jaw hadn't grown as much as the top jaw. When she came to see me, she told me, "I've lived with this bite and crooked teeth my whole life, and I've always wanted to straighten my teeth. But when I first saw an orthodontist back when I was twenty-five, he told me I needed braces and jaw surgery—and I didn't want surgery." He insisted that she needed it, though, so she didn't go back for treatment. Ten years later, she went to another orthodontist and got the same plan, and ten years after that, a third orthodontist gave her the same prognosis and recommendation. But now she was wondering if something else could be done for her.

After I did Delia's exam, I told her that I agreed with the evaluation of a skeletal discrepancy, and that, yes, she could benefit from jaw surgery. But I also understood that she didn't want that, so an alternative plan would be to align her teeth and leave the skeletal discrepancy as it was, meaning, the bite would stay as it was, which was fine since she did not have any issues resulting from it, and the alignment of her teeth would be great. Her smile would be beautiful, and it would be much easier to keep her teeth clean and her gums healthy over time. She was delighted! When we offer an alternative plan, our main goal is to make sure patients are much better off than when they started while we're meeting their needs and wishes. Delia finished her treatment and she couldn't have been happier with her appearance. While it was not an ideal result from a textbook standpoint, it was beautiful and functional, which was everything she'd dreamed of, and she was very thankful that after having waited for so many years, she got what she'd always wanted.

Very often at these first appointments, the patient will ask, "Will I need to have teeth removed?" After all, nobody wants to get a tooth removed, and you do hear the stories about people having to have extractions as part of their orthodontic plan. At our office, we have a non-extraction treatment philosophy, meaning we will do everything we can to avoid taking a tooth out, so we very rarely have teeth extracted. We only recommend tooth extraction when its benefit is greater than not extracting. And, of course, all our patients secretly hold their breath until I say, "You don't need headgear!"

How long will your treatment take to complete? When you start, we will give you an estimated treatment time based on the time a case like yours typically takes to resolve. There are other things that will affect your treatment, though: how good you are about taking care of your teeth and following recommendations when it comes to elastics and aligner wear and taking care of your braces. The growth rate and pattern of children and teenagers can also have an impact on the length of a treatment. All that said, most cases range between twelve and twenty-four months of treatment. And we use the latest technology and treatment mechanics to ensure treatment will be as effective and short as possible, while achieving a great result.

How much will the treatment cost? We believe that high-quality treatment should be attainable by everyone. Our financial specialist will work with you to help maximize the benefit and help you tailor payment arrangements that are affordable to you. Many of our patients use a combination of orthodontic benefits, HSA or FSA, and our low down payment and interest-free options. We will file claims on your behalf, and we're both in-network and out-of-network providers. For a more complete discussion of fees and payment options, see chapter eight, titled "How Do I Pay for This?"

Patients always want to know if they will need to wear a retainer after finishing treatment. The answer is invariably yes. As we explain in chapter five, wearing your retainer every night will keep your results in place and looking beautiful. Failing to wear them will allow your teeth to move back to where they were and can mean you'll need to go through orthodontics again—and nobody wants that! It can happen quickly, too, so we offer a five-year warranty program which allows you to get as many retainers as needed for the first five years after treatment completion, and you may re-enroll in the program after five years for a fee less than the cost of a new retainer. As the end of treatment approaches, we will discuss what your options are so you can choose the type of retainer you think you'll do best with to ensure you can keep your beautiful results.

After your appointment, we send a letter to your dentist, along with copies of the images taken. In our letter, we outline our findings and recommendations for items such as wisdom teeth so we are all on the same page and working toward the same goal.

WHAT NEXT?

After you have had your initial questions answered (and we're more than happy to answer as many as you have!), your next question might well be, "When do I start?"

At that point, the financial coordinator will sit down with you and help you set up a payment plan that's comfortable for you. They will also help you with the paperwork so we can file claims for you.

After we agree on a plan you're comfortable with, we will schedule your next visit to deliver your aligners, put braces on, or deliver appliances, depending on what you have decided on.

The appointment to put braces on usually lasts about sixty to ninety minutes. This first installation appointment will be your longest during your treatment because we like to take our time to make sure things are precisely done. Please check chapter four, titled "Orthodontics 101," where we talk more about appliances.

Some parents wonder if their child has dental anxiety. Honestly, sometimes even adult patients don't like visiting the dentist. During this first visit, all we're going to do is take some x-rays, which are different from the x-rays the dentist takes. We don't have to put the film inside your mouth. With our machine, you just bite on a little stick and the machine itself rotates around your head, so there's virtually nothing inside your mouth. These are the most comfortable digital x-rays you can imagine. Also, we don't need to make molds of your teeth, which orthodontists used to do and which often cause anxiety because a lot of patients are gaggers or gag just from thinking about having something in their mouth.

Instead of taking old-fashioned impressions, we use a special scanner that takes a fancy series of photographs to produce a 3-D image of your teeth and bite, which helps us to make a really precise plan. This is almost like making a movie of your teeth. We have a small camera that goes in your mouth. The video it's taking goes up on the screen and creates that 3-D model of the teeth and the bite. For patients who have a small mouth or are not comfortable with having things in their mouth, we can take breaks, and it usually only takes about five to ten minutes to do a scan. In some cases we will also take photos of the teeth.

WORKING WITH THE FEARFUL CHILD

If, during the initial exam and consultation, we notice our young patients are a little nervous, we are extra careful to make them comfortable. When I see a young child for the first time, I determine whether that child can benefit from treatment and is developmentally ready for treatment. Orthodontists are trained—as are the treatment coordinators at our office—to read those clues. Our goal is to make children comfortable because we're going to be seeing them for many visits. So, even though I may decide that some children are ready for treatment at that first visit, I will spend time with them, explaining the plan to them in language they can understand, showing them videos of the appliances, and telling them what to expect. This really reassures them, enlists them as partners in their plan, and makes them far more compliant and comfortable with both the office environment and the team. When those children come back for the next appointment, they're primed on what to expect, and it goes much more easily.

Sometimes we see children who have such dental anxiety that they refuse to sit in the "patient chair" or open their mouth during the first visit. Our goal then becomes getting them comfortable with us, which generally involves having them come in for a few visits and doing a little bit during each appointment: taking photos, taking some measurements of their mouth, doing a scan, and so forth. Once they are comfortable, we start treatment.

Often, children are worried about pain. When I see children looking tense, I ask if they're afraid the procedure is going to hurt. If they say yes, I offer to show them my tools and explain how they work. And then I show them what we're going to do and ask them if that is okay. Nine times out of ten, that demonstration totally defuses the situation because now they understand what's going to happen and there's nothing to be afraid of. We are always careful to explain what's going to happen, even if it's something very obvious and simple to us, because, of course, it's not obvious to the child.

And we also design the treatment plan for those little patients, based on what we feel they can tolerate in their mouth. We're not going to put something in there that is very intrusive, such as an expander and top and bottom braces all at once. If they need an expander, we start with that. Then, when they come back, we'll put in the bottom braces. On their next visit, we'll put in the top braces. By doing one thing at a time, these young patients are not over-whelmed. We stage the treatment based on what we see they need and what's going to make them most comfortable.

ONCE YOUR BRACES ARE ON …

Once your braces are on, we go over instructions on how to care for the braces, and how to keep your teeth and gums healthy. We give you tips on foods to avoid, and how you can help get your finished results faster. We let you know what to expect in terms of discomfort (most people get over any initial discomfort in a few days) and getting used to the braces. Adults generally take a little longer than children to get comfortable with their braces, but within a week, they'll be used to them.

If you're getting started with Invisalign, your aligners will be delivered about one month after the initial exam. That allows your doctor enough time to detail and customize the tooth movements that are going to be delivered by the aligners, and to get the aligners fabricated. Your Invisalign delivery appointment will take thirty minutes to an hour, depending on your case.

In our practice, on the day you come to get your braces or Invisalign delivered, we give you a written treatment plan.

When you come in to get started with the treatment, you'll also get a treatment plan letter, which explains the orthodontic issues, the goals of our treatment, the plan on how we are going to get there, and the estimated treatment time. We find that giving our patients all this in writing helps us assure them we are all on the same page.

WE UNDERSTAND IT'S A FAMILY MATTER

Sometimes, after parents visit us with their child, they want to go home and talk with their spouse before making any decisions about payment plans or treatment for their child. We get it. This is a big step and one you need to be clear about, going forward. To make it easy for you, we'll send you a link to a calculator program that you can play with at home. It lets you try out different down-payment amounts and monthly payments so you can figure out what works for you. Once you've arrived at a plan that suits your needs and your budget, you click a button that sends that information to us, and we'll proceed with setting up your next appointment.

When a child is examined, sometimes we determine that although we can see a problem down the line, it's too soon for orthodontic intervention. When that's the case, we monitor the child to determine the best timing to get started. At that point we'll enroll the child in our Growth Guidance program, and will see your child every six months to monitor jaw growth and tooth eruption and determine the best time to get started. This service is complimentary until your child is ready to start treatment. We view the Growth Guidance program as a time to get to know your family, as well as your child's growth and treatment needs, which leads to better, more efficient results when we are ready to begin.

OUR GOAL? WHITE GLOVE SERVICE FOR YOU, EVERY STEP OF THE WAY

We want every patient to have a great experience, from that very first phone call all the way to getting the retainers. Every process, every team member, every step in the journey is focused on that goal. Our systems are designed to make sure there are no loose ends and our patients' questions, concerns, and needs are addressed. Everyone who comes through our door can expect the best treatment and the best results possible and feel welcome, valued, and appreciated. The fact is, we really care how our patients feel. We're here for them, and we're constantly fine-tuning the way we do things to make sure their experience is as good as it can be, and that our patients are delighted with their results. We love what we do, and it shows.

CHAPTER ONE

—

Orthodontic Myths Busted

by Dr. Giannetti

A big part of my job is busting myths, the mistaken assumptions and misinformation that sometimes scare people away from getting the work they need. Where do these mistaken ideas come from? Part of the problem is that the Internet, while a valuable tool for research, is also full of confusingly written or just plain incorrect information. People are often hearing these myths from friends or relatives and accepting them as facts. Other times, they themselves were in braces many years ago, and they're expecting that their child's experience now will be the same as theirs was. But that's not true. For example, I'll tell the parents that the child's braces will need to be on for one to two years, and they're astonished that their teeth can be aligned so quickly, saying things like, "Wow! I had to wear them for three years. Are you sure you can move them that fast?" Another instance would be when a parent brings her seven-year-old in for a screening because the dentist told her she should, and she is surprised when I tell her we don't need to start orthodontic treatment yet. Instead, we are going to monitor the child's growth and start when the timing is perfect.

It makes sense. We all make assumptions about the world and how things work based on our own experiences. Just like the rest of medicine, orthodontics has also come a long way very quickly, and many of those notions don't hold true anymore. I'm sure family doctors are doing things differently than they were in 1985. At least, I hope so! The orthodontic field has a similarly robust scientific community constantly engaged in research and publishing. As a matter of fact, one of the things you have to do to graduate from your orthodontic residency is original research. It's quite challenging to get into an orthodontic program in the first place. You've got to go through dental school for a start, which is no easy feat, and only a tiny percentage of those graduates who apply—about 10 percent—are subsequently accepted into orthodontics programs. For the most part, people who are orthodontists are smart, and they're driven. They care about their profession. When a patient comes in with a problem, they want to solve it. That's driven the pace of change, and those changes are why much of what you believe about orthodontics is probably wrong.

Let's bust some of the most persistent myths and misconceptions that surround orthodontics.

MYTH #1
"Adults Can't Get Braces"

This is one I still hear, even though many adults are in treatment today. This misconception comes from people's experiences twenty-five years ago. In the '90s, it was relatively rare to treat adults with orthodontics. Science, technology, and experience has expanded so much that we're able to do things we didn't realize were possible back then.

Today's adults are more interested in keeping their youthful appearance than their parents were, and many of them, members of the baby boomer generation, weren't able to get treatment as children. As they got older and their own children left home, they began to ask for treatment to give them the smiles they'd always wanted. Orthodontists adapted: they did the research and the problem solving to make sure that they could serve that patient population, and subsequently, the demand for adult treatment is growing every year. When I was in my residency program between '95 and '98, I enjoyed treating adults, and I focused on that aspect of my education. I knew I wanted to serve adults, and I saw that the demand was there. When I bought this practice in 2001, I bought it from an orthodontist who didn't accept adults as patients. In our practice today, 50 percent of our patients are adults.

How old can you be and still get treatment? Honestly, there's no ceiling. So far, the oldest patient I've treated was eighty-five, and I have many people in their late seventies and early eighties in treatment at any given time.

That eighty-five-year-old didn't initially come in for aesthetic reasons; she had fallen and broken her jaw, and when it healed, her teeth no longer fit together properly, so she couldn't chew her food. She had spoken to another orthodontist, and the message she got there was effectively, "Well, you're going to be dead soon, so just get used to soft food. Why would you want to spend years straightening your teeth?" That wasn't good enough for her, and rightly so. She told me, "I just need to eat real food again. I don't know how long I'm going to live, but I'm still a person, and I don't want to lose that part of my life."

I agreed. Who wants to live on soft food if there is an option? We did braces for her for about a year, and she was a perfect patient and a pleasure to treat. When we finished, her smile was amazing. Seeing a photo of her teeth, you'd swear she wasn't over forty. And her bite was fully functional, which meant no more soft foods. She was delighted with the results, and she's still enjoying them.

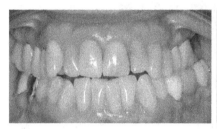 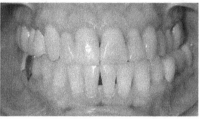

Before and after treatment for our eighty-year-old patient.

MYTH #2:
"Children Don't Need to See an Orthodontist until Their Adult Teeth Are All Nearly In"

This is a persistent myth, and a harmful one, because, in fact, there's a lot of good we can do for some children between six and nine years of age who have a jaw that's not growing properly and needs correcting. When children are young and their jaws are growing and more flexible, expanding their jaw or palate is a much easier thing to do than it is in adulthood, when surgery may be required. For a fuller explanation of when and why early treatment is indicated, read chapter three about phase 1 treatment. For now, please believe me when I tell you that there's sound science behind the American Association of Orthodontists' recommendation that an orthodontist should screen your child at no later than seven years of age. I see children literally every day who—either because of genetics or habits such as thumb sucking and tongue thrusting—have issues that need to be addressed. And while most children won't need phase 1 treatment, those who do can benefit from it enormously.

A family recently brought two of their children into our office for that early screening because their dentist had suggested it; I recommended phase 1 treatment for both of them. The parents could see the developing problem with one of the children and agreed to put her in treatment. But the other's issues weren't as obvious, and they wondered if they could just wait until she was older. I knew that the first child was going to have a big problem down the road if we didn't address it now, so we started her treatment, but in her sister's case, we decided to wait since she was borderline. Then, about three or four months later, the parents said, "We are so impressed and amazed at how Michelle's treatment is going that we want to know if it's too late or if it's still okay to treat her sister. We had told you that we wanted to wait, but now we understand what you were saying because we can see it in Michelle."

I was delighted they'd come around because it meant that Michelle's sister would have a much easier time overall since she was young enough for biology to still be on our side. They both got expanders, and the problems were corrected.

MYTH #3:
"I'll Be the Only Adult in a Room Full of Children at the Orthodontist's Office"

That's just no longer the case, and if you're an adult who wants and needs orthodontic treatment, you should look for a practice in which the orthodontist sees a lot of adults, because there are differences in how treatment is done.

Treatment for an adult is very different from treatment for a child. For example, removing teeth is a standard practice many orthodontic offices; and the orthodontist uses the space created to align the teeth. But in an adult, removing teeth has a lot of risks associated with it, and adult gums and bone don't respond the same way as teenage bone and gums. So, if you treat an adult as you would a teenager, you could wind up with compromised results. That's why, as an adult, you need an orthodontist with extensive experience of treating adults.

Adults need a practitioner who is willing and able to explain what is happening to them at any stage of treatment, whereas most teenagers have no interest in the process. As an adult, you are entitled to get clear and appropriately nontechnical explanations for everything that your orthodontist is doing or proposing to do, and your questions should be welcome and answered thoroughly.

If you really don't want to be there when the children are, try to set your appointments at times other than between 3:30 and 5:30 p.m., since that's when offices get the bulk of their younger patients. Most of our adult patients come in in the morning, so for the most part, our mornings are full of adults, and our afternoons are full of children. We see a lot of our adults during their lunch hour, too, because after braces are installed or aligners are fitted, check-ups are usually very quick and easy.

MYTH #4:

"I'll Be in Braces for at Least Three Years"

Good news for those of you who've avoided braces because you just couldn't face the prospect of having them for so long: The time it takes us now to straighten teeth has been shortened considerably. While a few more complex cases might take longer, most cases that would have taken three years in the past can be done now in two years or less. Why? Improved materials and technology have made orthodontics faster and more comfortable.

The technology of brackets—those devices that attach to your teeth, and to which we attach your braces—has improved, and we now use brackets that are better in terms of comfort, how

Improved materials and technology have made orthodontics faster and more comfortable.

efficiently they move teeth, and how often you need to come in for appointments. The wires are more flexible than the old steel wires of the past and get quicker results also. But don't lose sight of the fact that no matter what technology your orthodontist is investing in, the bottom line in terms of results will always be that orthodontist's skills and ability.

My feeling is that the best orthodontists will gravitate to the best available materials even though they cost more, because they give superior results. There are hundreds of kinds of wires and brackets on the market at all price points. They're all just tools. But in the hands of an experienced and highly skilled orthodontist, those tools will give you a faster and better result, with less pain and discomfort along the way. A less skilled practitioner could buy all the technology and the most expensive brackets on the market, but the results aren't necessarily going to be as good. The thing is that while the work of moving teeth is mechanical, experience and training matter a lot, as does the orthodontist's artistic vision of how the teeth should look at the end of treatment.

MYTH #5:
"All Orthodontists Do the Same Thing, So It Doesn't Really Matter Where You Go"

Not true! The fact is that ten orthodontists looking at the same patient will come up with ten different treatment plans, because there are always multiple ways to treat a case. Part of that is how we're educated: We're trained to look at every case from different angles and come up with multiple solutions to any problem. Then, as we gain more experience as practitioners, we develop techniques we feel give us the best results. For example, I only rarely recommend extractions because my experience has shown me that the results are not as good. So when crowding's an issue, I look for alternatives to solve the problem.

People are, understandably, confused by all these different opinions. Sometimes, when a prospective patient comes in for a consultation, I'll be the third orthodontist they've seen because they saw one they didn't really feel comfortable with, so they saw another one, who gave them a completely different treatment plan. When they come to me for a third opinion, they're flummoxed: how could there be more than one "right" way?

I always tell them, "I don't even want to know what somebody else said to you. I just want to tell you what I think. After I tell you what I think, you can tell me what they said, or you can ask me questions." I love it when people get multiple opinions because I think I'm good at explaining and justifying the treatment plans that I suggest. It doesn't surprise me that they've gotten different opinions, because orthodontic training and experience varies, and educational programs differ.

A patient recently come into my office for a consultation, and I told him I could correct his problem with either Invisalign or with braces. It was his choice. He was shocked. He said his general dentist did Invisalign treatments and told him they wouldn't work for him. I explained that perhaps his dentist didn't feel his case was within his personal comfort zone, but I was experienced and confident it would work since I had performed this type of treatment successfully on many patients. It is just another tool in my toolbox.

In choosing an orthodontist, be sure you're comfortable with the treatment plan, the practitioner, and the office environment, because you're going to be a regular visitor for some time. Orthodontics is usually a long-term relationship.

MYTH #6:
"I'd Have to Come to the Office Every Three Weeks and I Don't Have the Time"

Good news: you don't have to visit the office as often anymore. Back in the '80s patients had office check-ups every three weeks. But nowadays, depending on where you are in your treatment plan and your orthodontist's preferences, it's likely that you will only need to schedule an appointment every couple of months.

MYTH #7:

"Once I've Got My Braces, I Don't Really Need to Come in for All Those Visits Because They Work by Themselves"

While we may wish that braces were "set it and forget it," that's not the case. Remember: braces are just a tool, and unless someone's working on them and making the necessary adjustments, they're not going to do their job.

Let's say you come into our office, and we tell you, "We don't need to see you for ten weeks." That's because the treatment we just did for you will work for ten weeks. But after ten weeks, we will need to make the adjustments that will keep the treatment working. It's not just what's in your mouth that straightens your teeth; it's the people who are making the adjustments and following the treatment plan that's been created for you.

In our practice, we lay out all the appointments when we agree on the treatment plan so our patients know they have a set number of appointments to get to the finish line and are aware of where they are on the timeline.

MYTH #8:

"Braces Are Ugly"

Another one we can put to rest! Modern braces are a far cry from the steely grille you may have had as a young teen. Today's braces are much more aesthetic, and some are virtually invisible. Clean, shiny metal braces are quite attractive (I know I may be a little biased!). And clear braces are also available. They are made of either porcelain or plastic, although we don't use the plastic ones in our practice, because they tend to stain over time and that's not so pretty. The porcelain braces are guaranteed not to stain and are see-through because porcelain is glass, so they're aesthetically acceptable.

Invisalign aligners are a great option for a lot of people. They are clear plastic trays, and because you put a new one on every week, they don't have time to get discolored.

Because more and more adults are getting braces, there's really not the stigma there used to be about having braces or wanting to do something to improve your smile. When I first started doing Invisalign in 2001, an older lady came to me. "I want my teeth to be straighter and my smile to look better," she said. "I heard there's this new thing called Invisalign and I don't want to have braces. Can you make it look better? I don't care if it's perfect. What matters most to me is that my friends at church don't know that I'm straightening my teeth." Clearly, she was worried about feeling judged, but attitudes have improved a lot since then—and so has Invisalign. She was delighted with her results, and nobody knew she'd had aligners.

MYTH #9:
"I Can't See an Orthodontist without a Referral"

You are free to make an initial appointment with whichever orthodontist you want. At your new-patient appointment, they will tell you what your insurance benefit is. You don't need to get a referral from your general dentist or anybody else.

MYTH #10:

"Braces Hurt"

Braces aren't supposed to hurt. If they do hurt, it's likely that something's not right and needs to be fixed. You should let your orthodontist take care of it.

But if your teeth are sore, that's normal, particularly at the start of treatment. Your teeth have to get sore to move, but the level of discomfort is minimal compared to what it used to be years ago. Why? Because the force levels that we use on people's teeth now are a hundred times less than the forces that were used twenty-five years ago.

> **The force levels that we use on people's teeth now are a hundred times less than the forces that were used twenty-five years ago.**

I know because I myself just had braces; Dr. Booms treated me in 2017! I had a fairly minor issue, but I thought, *You know what? I'm going to have braces. I can experience it from a patient's point of view so I can be sure that what I tell them is correct.* I'd had them before, back in 1983, and the difference in how comfortable these were in 2017 was night and day. I occasionally had to take some Tylenol or ibuprofen, but that was all I needed, a big difference from the experience I'd had in braces at the age of fifteen. Because of my experience, I am currently treating Dr. Booms.

MYTH #11:

"My Orthodontist Told Me Years Ago That I Couldn't Be Treated"

That may have been true back then, but our new techniques and technology mean that we can treat a lot of cases successfully that couldn't have been treated years ago. My advice would be to get a second opinion now, because the news may be good, and if it's not, get another opinion. If two or three good orthodontists tell you that you can't be helped, you may have to accept that. But don't go by what you were told in the past, even just five years ago, because things really have changed.

I have patients who come in for braces and when I ask them whether they want regular braces or Invisalign, many tell me, "I was told ten years ago I'm not an Invisalign case, so I'm fine having braces."

When I look into their mouths, I can tell them, "You're an easy Invisalign case. Would you like to have Invisalign?"

The response is always, "Really? Why did they tell me that ten years ago?" It's not that their practitioner back then was necessarily wrong; it's just that the technology has moved so quickly we can treat all kinds of cases that wouldn't have been possible to do in the past.

And even if you really can't be treated now, don't lose hope! In five or ten years, chances are good that the science will have advanced so much that you'll be treatable at that point.

MYTH #12:
"I Can't Afford Orthodontics"

Of course, orthodontic treatment isn't cheap. With the office overhead costs, educational costs, materials used, and so many other costs a practice has to cover, you do pay a fairly sizable amount, which may seem out of your reach.

But the majority of orthodontic offices will work with you to craft a payment plan that allows you to pay a fixed amount per month, and don't charge you any interest to finance your treatment, which puts treatment within the reach of most people. Certainly, in our practice, we want you to get the help you need and will do all we can to make it affordable. Our average patient pays between $100 and $200 per month.

Most of us make monthly payments for all kinds of things: cell phone service, cable, Netflix subscriptions, and so forth. If money's the big worry for you, talk to the person at your orthodontist's practice whose job it is to help you with financing. You'll probably be pleasantly surprised at how helpful that person can be. And remember that unlike your cable bill, orthodontics is an investment, one that will pay dividends for a lifetime for you or your child.

MYTH #13:
"I Heard That Braces Will Set Off the TSA Metal Detectors at the Airport"

I can speak from personal experience on this one: they definitely don't! I honestly don't know why. My earrings always do, but my braces didn't. Last year, when I was in metal braces, I flew on at least four different occasions and never set off the alarms when I went through the security check.

I hope I've busted whatever misconceptions you might have had, but remember that if you have any questions, orthodontists love to answer them, so don't hesitate to ask. You'll most likely be reassured by the answers.

—

CHAPTER TWO

Your Bite: How It Got That Way, and Why It Matters

by Dr. Giannetti

K ara's mom couldn't see much wrong with her daughter's teeth and told me so after our initial exam. "They look pretty straight to me. Does she really need braces?"

I showed her the x-rays and explained, "When Kara brings her front teeth together, she actually can't incise things—in other words, she can't bite properly. Have you ever noticed that she avoids biting down on food with her front teeth? Or maybe, when she eats a sandwich, she leaves the lettuce on the plate?"

At that point, Kara spoke up. "Yes, I do leave the lettuce! And I don't eat anything I'd have to bite off with my front teeth in public, because I can't." Her mom looked astonished. Why hadn't she ever mentioned it? Kara shrugged. "I thought you knew."

This kind of miscommunication is much more common than you might think, because so often we parents miss what's right in front of us, and our children don't bother to tell us, because it's just the way things have always been, so it's no big deal. When most people think about reasons for orthodontic treatment, they're thinking about the problems you can easily see—protruding teeth or teeth that overlap each other, for instance. But every bit as important is the bite, and while problems with your bite aren't always as evident, they do have consequences.

You wouldn't necessarily associate something such as persistent headaches with a bad bite, but in fact, when one of my patients reported having frequent headaches, it turned out that her bite was among the causes, and an imbalance of musculature, because the muscles of the face, the head, and the neck will compensate to get the teeth together.

Your temporomandibular joint (TMJ) that connects your lower jaw to your head is similar to a ball and socket joint, like your knee. If the joint is in the socket and the muscles are relaxed when your teeth come together but your teeth don't fit properly, your brain senses a problem. Then, the muscles engage and move the joint out of the socket in order to get your teeth together to function as best they can under the circumstances.

It's important to remember that everything in your body is connected: your cervical spine, your neck, your head, the muscles that connect your neck and your head, your tongue, TMJ, and your teeth. That's why if one thing is off, it's going to have an impact on the functionality and health of all the other parts.

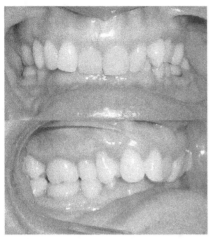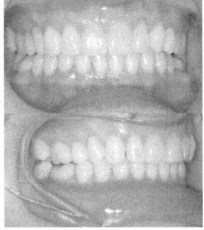

Before and after of an adult patient who had a severe overbite causing TMJ problems. The patient reported that her overbite got worse with age and when she was a child she didn't need orthodontics.

THE CASCADE OF PROBLEMS TAKES TIME TO DEVELOP

I see this frequently in both adults and children. In children, it's easily corrected. Usually, they don't have symptoms because they are very resilient. But when adults have that kind of issue and it's been present throughout their life, we start to see damage: persistent headaches, head and neck pain, and then, ultimately, cracking and breaking teeth. The condition often goes undiagnosed until, all of a sudden, things start to fall apart in their mouths. Typically, what I'll hear is, "I had one tooth crack and it broke and I lost it. And then I had another one, and three years later I had four of them. Now, all of a sudden, everything is just falling apart."

That's because once we get past a certain threshold of issues in our body, whether that's inflammation, pain, or TMJ, we start to see a cascade of problems, and it's very difficult to get back to the state of health where we were prior to hitting that limit.

Possibly, when the previous patient was twelve years old, he had a moderate overbite, but his teeth looked straight enough, and his parents shrugged it off. But as he grew, the disequilibrium became increasingly worse, until something traumatic happened to bring it to a head. Maybe he was hit in the mouth and his front tooth was broken, or he cracked a tooth in the back of his mouth. Perhaps he'd been clenching and grinding over time. Then, in his middle age, all of those things start adding up, and he passed over that threshold where everything starts falling apart.

Now, this patient loses a tooth, so he goes to the dentist. But because his bite's not optimal, the dentist can't really fix the tooth in a predictable way. So that tooth replacement is compromised, which adds to the compromise that was already going on, and then something else happens, and that leads to another tooth being cracked. It's a snowball effect until that person finally goes to an orthodontist and gets that bad bite corrected. I see probably four or five adults with this kind of problem every day.

Recently, a fifty-year-old man, Larry, came in to see me. He'd been to his dentist because of a cracked tooth and had mentioned, "For some reason, my front teeth are really short and are cracking. Can we do something about that? I don't really remember them being ever short when I look back at pictures of myself, and I can see that there's a lot of wear on my teeth."

The dentist told him, "Yes, you've worn the enamel away and now we can see the dentin showing through your teeth because you've had this overbite your whole life and you've ground it away. Before we replace this tooth, you need to have braces in order to fix your bite." That's how Larry ended up in our office. Because he cared about his health and he wanted to keep his teeth, he decided to have braces. When he was done with his braces he got the tooth replaced, and he also got veneers on his front teeth to bring them back to the size they were when he was younger, and to keep them from wearing down further. Once the soft dentin under the hard enamel is exposed, subsequent wear of the teeth is accelerated. The same thing had happened to his wife, and I ended up treating them both.

It's worth noting that both of them had been very meticulous about their oral care throughout their lives. They had routinely gone to the dentist. They both had very good jobs as attorneys and had dental insurance, yet the problem simply hadn't made itself obvious. It's just that they'd both hit the age of crossing that threshold, so all of a sudden, things began falling apart and they had to do something about it.

BAD BITE AND GUM RECESSION

Gum recession is another problem that can be caused by a bad bite. Teeth sit in the bone and the gum, so when there's constant traumatic force on the teeth, the bone responds, as does the gum tissue that covers it. Not only can you get gum recession, but you can also get bone loss around the teeth.

> When your bite is good, your teeth fit together properly and can take the pressure. When the bite is bad, the force is distributed unequally, putting too much pressure on particular teeth.

What creates all this havoc? In a word, force—about 170 pounds' worth of force (on average) put on your molars when you bite down. When your bite is good, your teeth fit together properly and can take the pressure. When the bite is bad, the force is distributed unequally, putting too much pressure on particular teeth. They can only withstand that for so long.

WHAT YOU EAT IS ALSO TIED TO YOUR BITE

I mentioned Kara, my young patient who deliberately set aside any lettuce in a sandwich because she couldn't bring her teeth together well enough to bite through it. That might seem like a minor annoyance, but for people with significantly bad bites, it does affect how they masticate their food, as well as the types of foods they tend to eat.

Some people can only eat soft food because of their bites. They might avoid hard or crisp foods, and unfortunately, these categories include healthy things our bodies need, such as fresh fruits and vegetables. Not surprisingly, their overall health suffers. That's true with children too. More than once, I've fixed a child's bad bite so that the jaw was no longer shifting out of the socket and the teeth could come together properly, only to have the parent come back to me after treatment and confide, "I had no idea. I just thought he hated apples and carrots!" Now that the bite was corrected and comfortable, the child discovered the pleasure of biting into a juicy apple.

WHAT CAUSES A BAD BITE?

The most common culprit is genetics, which determine how your jaw and bite will develop. If bad bites run in your family, you're very likely to have the same problem. Once genetics have determined what an infant is going to start out with in life, the environment takes over. There are a lot of environmental causes of bad bites. One is prolonged thumb sucking or the use of pacifiers. Another is a habitual tongue thrust, or mouth breathing.

Mouth breathing, or the inability to breathe through the nose, can be a major cause of growth-related bite problems. This happens to a lot of children who have precursors to sleep disordered breathing, such as enlarged tonsils or adenoids, or allergies. To illustrate this, in the '70s, studies were done in which researchers plugged the nasal cavities of monkeys and let them grow and adapt to not being able to breathe through their noses.[1] The results were quite dramatic. Their faces got noticeably longer because they had to breathe through their mouth. Their palates got higher. Their arches got narrower. They developed what to this day orthodontists call "adenoid facies," which we correlate with people whose enlarged adenoids and tonsils blocked their airways in childhood and persisted throughout their growth and development.

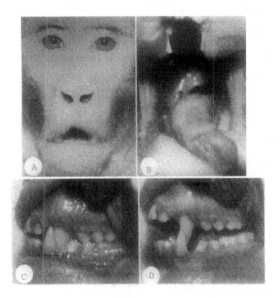

Another environmental cause can be the physical traumas that most children experience when they're growing up. Maybe they fell on the coffee table and knocked a baby tooth out. The buds of the permanent teeth grow right underneath the roots of the baby teeth, so sometimes, trauma to a baby tooth can dislodge or move the developing bud of the permanent tooth, which eventually comes in crooked.

1   EP Harvold et al., "Primate experiments on oral respiration," *Am J Orthod.* 79, no. 4 (April 1981): 359–72, https://www.ncbi.nlm.nih.gov/pubmed/6939331.

I've seen patients whose teeth came in rotated over ninety degrees or in a completely different spot than where they were supposed to be. For example, two teeth can flip places in a transposition.

Cavities are another environmental cause of a bad bite. When children get cavities that cause their baby teeth to crack or be lost, if the baby tooth isn't fixed or a space maintainer is not put in, the teeth just drift around. An analogy I use with my patients is that when you get on a crowded bus, everyone shifts a little to make room. But when someone gets off, everyone shifts again to get themselves a little more space. They don't just leave that empty space empty, which is exactly what your teeth do. In fact, teeth grow until they touch another tooth and this process can be the root of most problems when it comes to environmental causes.

HOW CAN A BITE BE REPAIRED?

Orthodontists are specialists in repairing bad bites. Depending on the specifics of the case and the age of the patient, treatment could be something as simple as an expander for a child, or full braces in an adult. For a seven-year-old whose jaw is shifting out of the socket because the upper teeth don't meet the lower teeth, we can install an expander and solve the problem. No braces are necessarily required. The issue is resolved in three months, and the expander is removed in six months. Again, getting your child examined at an early age by an orthodontist can uncover a problem such as a bad bite before it causes damage and becomes harder to fix.

Remember Kara? She got an expander and within a year, her bite was fine. My older patient, Larry, was treated with full braces and did very well with them. It took two years, and now, he has his veneers, his implant, and a wonderful smile—and he wears his retainer every night!

"CAN I GET ORTHODONTIC TREATMENT IF I HAVE GUM DISEASE?"

Yes, you can. In, fact, I regularly get referrals from a periodontist who is a gum specialist. He sends me adult patients who have a history of periodontal disease that is now controlled, such as chronic bone loss and gum problems, because he's worried about them losing their teeth due to incorrect forces from a bad bite. Putting braces on someone with a history of gum disease seems counterintuitive to most people because they believe that, due to their bone loss and weak gums, orthodontics will make their situation worse. But it actually makes their situation better. By the time we're halfway through their orthodontic treatment, and even while they are still in treatment, their gum health is already much improved because we're putting their teeth in the right place. When they're done with treatment, the long-term prognosis for their teeth is better.

One woman came to our office for a second opinion after an orthodontist had told her she wasn't a good candidate for braces because she was going to lose her teeth, and moving them would make them fall out more quickly. We explained to her that the way we move teeth, with low forces, would actually decrease, rather than increase, the inflammation. And it did. When we were done, her periodontist couldn't believe how healthy her gums were. Now he sends us a lot of his patients.

If you're seeing abnormal wear on your teeth, or if you're experiencing any kind of jaw pain, tooth pain, or other symptoms your dentist can't find a good reason for, get an exam and assessment from an orthodontist. The underlying problem may well be your bite, and the sooner you get it fixed, the less damage you'll have to repair in the future.

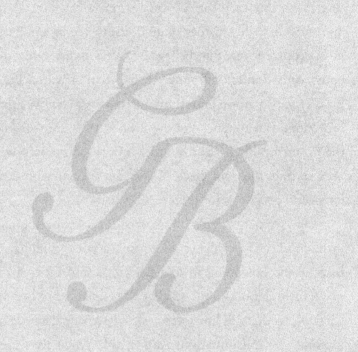

CHAPTER THREE

Phase 1 Treatment:
Why Your Young Child May Need Orthodontic Intervention

by Dr. Booms

As the science of orthodontics has advanced, so has our understanding of how our jaws and face grow, and our ideas about when to treat have changed too. Years ago, orthodontists counseled patients to wait until all their permanent teeth had come in to treat, which was typically about age twelve. But today, it's common to treat a seven-year-old, and that's creating some understandable confusion among parents, particularly those who had orthodontics themselves back in the days when dentists didn't recommend treatment until the early teen years.

The American Association for Orthodontists recommends that every child be screened by an orthodontist by age seven. Why? Seven is when most children have their first permanent molars and incisors so we can evaluate whether the jaws are growing normally, whether or not the teeth are coming in properly, and if there's enough room for permanent teeth as they come in.

Most children will not need any intervention at this stage, but it's critical to identify those who do. If something isn't growing normally, biology is on the patient's side when the patient is still young, growing, and developing. The top jaw (the maxilla) has soft spots when the child is younger, which will eventually harden to interlock with the rest of the jaw, much like the soft spots on a baby's skull. When the top jaw is still soft, it's more malleable, and it's far easier to mold and change its growth at that stage. Once the patient is an adult and those soft spots have hardened into bone, treatment can still be accomplished, but the magnitude of change we can achieve without surgery decreases and may also not be as comfortable or as stable.

Orthodontists are experts on facial growth and prescribe treatment according to what can be accomplished at different stages of development. That is why it is key to be seen by an orthodontist at an early age, when growth can be redirected.

> Our family have been patients of Dr. Giannetti for fourteen years. Dr. Giannetti has given three of our children such beautiful smiles. She is very knowledgeable and we always felt 100 percent confident in our children's treatment plans. The staff at Dr. Giannetti's office has always been friendly and helpful. I refer to Dr. Giannetti as the "ortho goddess," but all jokes aside, she is hands down is the absolute best. I can't thank her enough for taking such great care of my kids all these years. Thanks a million,
>
> **Jennifer Pitts**

WHY IS EARLY TREATMENT CALLED PHASE 1?

Early treatment is referred to as phase 1 because most children who require early treatment will also benefit from a phase 2 treatment, usually when most of the permanent teeth have come in. The nature of phase 1 is typically more orthopedic, meaning that it's aimed at addressing a developing problem and changing the way the jaws are growing to bring things back to normal. Phase 2 is a dental phase in that we're dealing with the alignment of the teeth, and if needed, it will be done after most of the permanent teeth have come in. During phase 1, orthodontists are usually not too concerned with the alignment of the teeth. At this point, we're more concerned that the teeth are coming in as they should be and the jaws are growing properly.

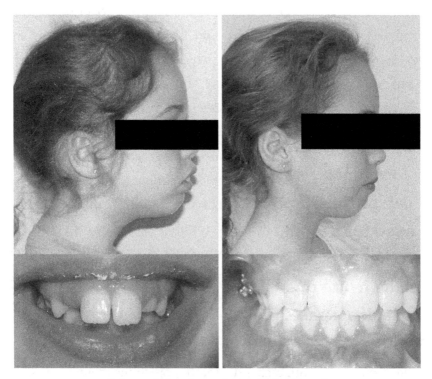

Before and after photos demonstrating Phase 1
treatment with an expander and braces.

WHAT WE SCREEN FOR WHEN EXAMINING YOUNG CHILDREN

When I'm doing an exam on a younger child, there are four main things I'm looking for: **crowding**, **crossbite**, what's called a **class three**, and **oral habits**.

Crowding occurs when there is not enough room for a tooth to come in, so those new teeth may become impacted and unable to find their way into their proper places in the mouth. When they do erupt, they come in far out of alignment. If, at this early stage, I can identify a crowding issue, I can proactively create space where it's needed to allow the teeth to come in naturally where they belong. This is easiest to do when the child is still growing, because the gums and the bone respond in a healthy, predictable, and favorable way. By doing phase 1 treatment, we can prevent the need for a tooth to be extracted in the future due to lack of space. Crowding in growing children may mean that their arches need to be developed or expanded to make enough space to accommodate all the teeth, a process that's much easier and faster at this age than it would be for an adult.

> By doing phase 1 treatment, we can prevent the need for a tooth to be extracted in the future due to lack of space.

Crowding causes other issues too. If a tooth comes in too far to the outside, for instance, it's coming out of the bone where the gum is relatively thin. That means that even if we make space and bring the tooth down later, the thin gum around the tooth makes the tooth more prone to gum recession over time. If we see it early and make space, that tooth will come up in the center of the bone, surrounded by nice thick gum, and will be less likely to have recession in the long run than if we'd let it come all the way to the outside and then moved it back.

A **crossbite** means one or more of the top teeth are biting into the inside of the bottom teeth. Sometimes when children have a crossbite of the back teeth, they need to shift the jaw to one side to be able to chew, creating what we call a functional shift.

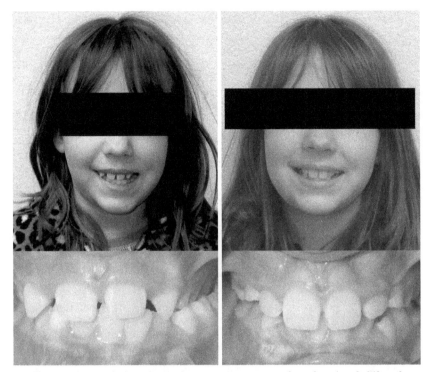

These before and after photos demonstrate treatment for a functional shift and crossbite. The before picture is notable for her chin being deviated to the left and how her face is crooked. The treatment was accomplished with only an expander.

A functional shift creates issues in the mouth of growing children because if they're constantly shifting the bottom jaw to one side to be able to chew, the jaw will adapt by growing in that direction in the long term. In the short term, the jaw joint is dislocating out of the socket every time they eat. If they spend their growth years with this functional shift uncorrected, it can result in an asymmetric jaw in adulthood. Again, this is easier to rectify in a young child, when the crossbite can be corrected and brought back to normal with appliances.

Typically, a crossbite is corrected by means of appliances (expander on the top jaw or braces). This eliminates the crossbite and also develops the jaw to make more room for permanent teeth to come in and for the tongue.

A **class three** issue happens when the bottom jaw grows more than the top jaw. In some children, this may result in an underbite, or a crossbite of the front teeth. For others, the teeth may compensate for the bottom jaw's growth by changing their angulation, which results in **camouflage discrepancy**: though the jaws are growing in this undesirable way, you don't actually see an underbite. That means that, as a parent, you won't see anything wrong, but your orthodontist can identify this growth pattern by analyzing the x-rays taken during the screening exam.

I can generally determine if this is the case just by talking to a child. If children do not show their upper front teeth when they smile, something is wrong. It is not normal to see a child's lower front teeth instead of their upper front teeth.

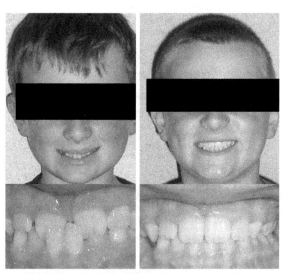

This before and after photo demonstrates a Class III malocclusion (underbite) and an anterior cross bite. Treatment was accomplished with Phase 1 braces. Notice how the lower teeth are showing in the before smiling photo, and after treatment, the upper teeth are more prominent.

It's very important to treat these cases when the jaws are still malleable. The typical treatment involves wearing headgear at home to add forward pull to the top jaw and improve the midface. Since the top jaw is still soft, a very light force applied to the outside can change its growth pattern to make it normal.

An adult with a severe underbite may require jaw surgery to correct it, so phase 1 treatment early on can be crucial in avoiding the need for a jaw surgery in the future. If phase 2 treatment is required down the road, it will be far easier.

When we screen for **oral habits**, we're looking for things such as thumb or finger sucking, and also for **dysfunctional muscle patterns**, like tongue thrust and mouth breathing. Any of these can create enough force in the mouth of a growing child to alter the normal growth of the jaws.

Parents may be aware of their child's finger or thumb sucking habit, but a dysfunctional muscle pattern such as tongue thrust is harder to see, and they may not know that their child is doing it. This habit can persist into adulthood too. To illustrate this, notice right now as you read this book where your tongue is sitting—is your tongue touching the roof of your mouth? Is the tip of the tongue behind your teeth? If you answered yes, then good news, your tongue is where it is supposed to be. Now, go ahead and swallow. Does your tongue press against the roof of your mouth and your teeth come together? If so, good news again.

If not, you may have a tongue thrust. It happens when the tongue is positioned in between the teeth while swallowing or at rest, instead of being placed in the roof of the mouth. Because people swallow multiple times in an hour, tongue thrust puts enough pressure on the teeth to change how the jaws grow and how the teeth come together. Typically, when patients with a tongue thrust habit bite down, their teeth don't come together in the area where they're putting their tongue, so they've got an open bite in that area. It's a very tricky habit. Even if we bring the teeth back together, if the patients still have that tongue habit, they'll push the teeth apart again, eventually. It's hard enough to change a habit we're aware of, so imagine having to stop doing something you're not aware of doing! Early intervention in childhood is so helpful because we can proactively correct that tongue thrusting habit and prevent the damage.

In treating tongue thrust, we typically employ myofunctional therapy, a specialized therapy that addresses muscle function and habits. Sometimes we also use an appliance that directs the tongue to where it should go. It's important to note here that a myofunctional therapist is not the same as a speech therapist and myofunctional therapy is not speech therapy (although a speech therapist can also be a myofunctional therapist). A myofunctional therapist evaluates the whole function of the mouth: how patients chew, breathe, how they use their lips and facial muscles, and how they use their tongue to swallow. For many cases of tongue thrust in children, we work with a combination of an appliance and myofunctional therapy, and we get great results.

Another dysfunctional oral habit that can affect growth is mouth breathing. In these cases, in addition to myofunctional therapy, we typically enroll other specialists, such as an ENT, to treat the child as a whole.

As a general rule, the longer the habit persists, the harder it is to eliminate it and the more time it has to affect facial growth. That is why we have a program for patients starting as young as five years old for habit cessation.

At this age, once the child agrees to quit, there are things that parents can do at home, such as putting a coat of a very sour-tasting nail polish on the thumbnail or wrapping their thumb in athletic tape as a reminder. We encourage children to stop their habit on their own, but if that doesn't work, we have a formal treatment that is kind and successful for most children. Just ask! As a last resort, if our "self-help" program doesn't work, we can place a thumb crib on the top teeth, which sits there as a reminder, so when they put their thumb there, they realize, "Oh, I'm not supposed to do this," and that usually does the trick.

Again, getting them to the orthodontist's office at an early age is key to success. If children with an oral habit are treated at an early age, the damage can be undone. By directing the forces back to normal and molding the jaw in the right way, they can go back to growing in a normal way. But if we don't see them until they're twelve years old, the damage is done because a ton of improper facial growth has occurred that has been molded by the habit.

BUILDING A HEALTHY FOUNDATION FOR GROWTH AND DEVELOPMENT

I like to compare phase 1 treatment to the first step in building a house, which is creating a solid foundation that includes normal muscle function. Phase 2 is done at around age twelve because most of the adult teeth are in by then. If we've got a good foundation—a well-developed jaw with enough room to accommodate the teeth— even if the teeth are not in good alignment, we are in good shape.

In evaluating whether or not a patient needs phase 2 treatment, we're looking for **crowding, class two**, and **canines**. At this age— usually around twelve—we can align the teeth and address significant **crowding** effectively, and most often without need for extractions.

In a **class two** patient, the bottom jaw is growing less than the top jaw. This is where an orthodontist's extensive training in jaw growth and development plays a big role in identifying the best time to treat different problems. When children are going through

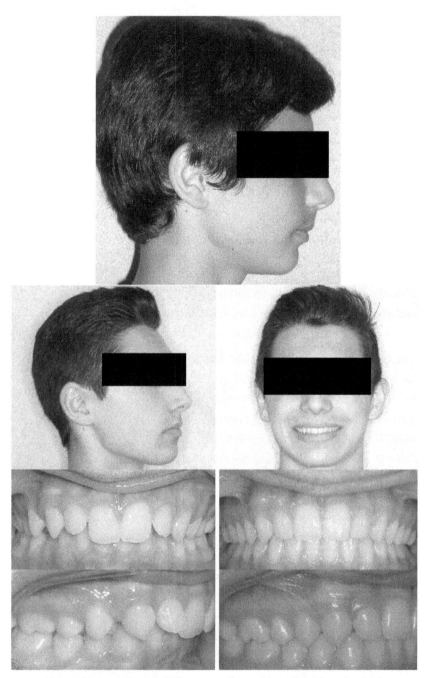

This patient was treated during a growth spurt to redirect the growth of his jaws. Braces and a functional appliance were used. Notice the profile before orthodontic treatment with the short bottom jaw (top picture) and the profile picture below it with a stronger chin and more proportional jaws.

a growth spurt, the bottom jaw grows a lot. If the bottom jaw is too short for the top jaw, we can use different techniques—appliances, braces with rubber bands, or Invisalign with rubber bands, for instance—to direct the bottom jaw and encourage it to grow even more than it's already growing to catch up with the top. Again, the patient's age and development is key to success. In an adult, a short bottom jaw can only be brought forward by jaw surgery, whereas if we see a twelve-year-old with a short bottom jaw, we can affect the jaw's growth enough to fix the bite and improve the profile and the jaw structure by directing their growth, which is much easier on the patient (see photos on facing page.)

Canines—also known as eye teeth on the top—often create problems coming in because they move along a fairly tortuous path to their correct position in the mouth. Sometimes they miss it and don't find their way which is called an **impaction**.

If you're just looking at the patient's mouth, you won't see it happening until it's too late and damage may already have occurred. When we're monitoring children on a regular basis, we're more likely to know in advance that teeth are becoming impacted, and we can take noninvasive steps to help them find their way. Usually, that means having their dentist remove baby teeth to open up that needed space, or alternatively, we put in an expander to make more room in the jaw for the teeth to come in. This approach has a 70 percent chance of success at avoiding the impaction.

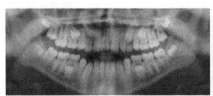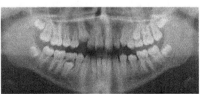

In the first image, the upper right canine is becoming impacted. By removing the baby tooth early, we opened up enough space for the canine tooth to grow in without an impaction, which you can see in the patient's x-ray one year later.

In cases where this approach doesn't prevent the impaction, we refer the patient to an oral surgeon who will surgically expose that tooth, and then we can guide that tooth into place with appliances. At our office, we have a 3-D x-ray machine that we use especially for those cases because a 2-D machine just doesn't offer the clarity and accuracy in seeing exactly where the tooth is. With 3-D imaging, we can create a very specific plan for the optimal mechanics to bring that tooth in without damaging the teeth around it.

How do we monitor children whose jaws may not be growing ideally? In our practice, we have what we call a Growth Guidance program, a free service we offer our patients and our referring dentists. This gives everyone piece of mind that we are being proactive but not overtreating. We never tell someone who brings in a seven-year-old that we don't see a problem now and "just come back when Susie is twelve." Beginning at age seven, we see patients about every six months to monitor their jaw growth and tooth eruption, so that small problems don't have a chance to turn into bigger ones. We take photos of their teeth at every appointment, examine the child's mouth, and take x-rays when they're needed. Should we find a problem developing—say an impacted tooth at age eleven, or a jaw not growing as much as it should—we're able to keep the issue from getting worse, spotting it when children are going through a growth spurt that might provide the best window in which to treat them. Sometimes people are surprised when we tell them this service is free, but, yes, it *is* free and we do not bill your insurance either. Why? The reason is that it is the right thing to do, and we care about our patients. Not many health care providers offer this type of service, but many orthodontists do.

The Growth Guidance program is something that we work really hard on because we believe it's a great benefit to our patients. No ethical orthodontists want to see their patients have any more treatment than is necessary.

WHEN AN ORTHODONTIST RECOMMENDS PHASE 1 TREATMENT …

Many parents are skeptical and highly suspicious of phase 1 treatment, because they think it's a scam to get younger children more treatment than they need. For all the reasons I've talked about above, that's just not the case—at least, not for most orthodontists. At our office, we recommend phase 1 treatment only when we're confident it will make phase 2 treatment shorter or more predictable, and/or the results better.

If you're not sure why your orthodontist is recommending phase 1, ask, "What will be the implications down the road if we opt not to do phase 1? Will it be less likely my child is going to have a good outcome down the road? Will it mean it's harder for her teeth to come in properly? Or will it significantly increase the length of treatment in phase 2?" Don't be afraid to ask for specifics. The fact is that most children don't need phase 1 treatment. But for those children who do, it's crucial that those parents know how and why their child can benefit from it.

Worried about choosing an orthodontist? Ask your dentist to recommend an orthodontist, because dentists are likely to know and trust the practitioners they recommend. Or ask your friends for a recommendation to an orthodontist they had a good experience with and do your research online. And if, at that initial exam, you have any doubts or any unanswered questions about what you're told, or if you're just not comfortable with the recommendations you get from that orthodontist, seek a second opinion.

Nearly every orthodontic practice will provide this kind of initial screening examination without any charge. Please don't fail to take your child in to be screened, because early intervention when it's needed is always the best way to go.

CASE STUDY: ALLIE

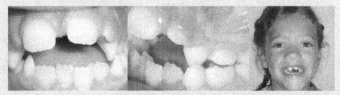

Before treatment.

Allie was only seven when her family dentist noticed that her tongue thrusting habit was causing her jaws to grow abnormally and told her mother that Allie needed to see an orthodontist. Mom was surprised. Surely age seven was too young for orthodontics? But that early intervention made it possible for me to correct the habit and change the growth pattern of her jaws so they'd be normal. That meant that by the time she was old enough for regular braces, all we needed to do was to align her teeth. We got a great result from phase 1 treatment. Phase 2 went very quickly and well because of that early treatment, and Allie's beautiful smile helped her to win a Miss Teen contest. Had her parents waited, she would certainly have required longer and more involved treatment, and the outcome would not have been nearly as good.

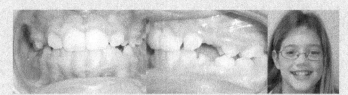

After Phase 1 treatment.

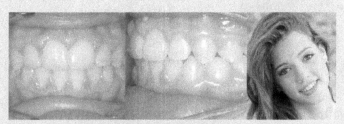

After Phase 2 treatment.

CHAPTER FOUR
———
Orthodontics 101

by Dr. Booms

I f you had braces as a child or even as a teenager, you're probably cringing at the memory of the separators, the bands, and those very tight wires. Fortunately, orthodontics has changed greatly, and the materials and techniques we use today are light-years from what was available even ten years ago. For instance, the wires we use are literally space-age—very flexible and far more comfortable than the stiff wires they replaced. At our office, we rarely use bands, so separators are no longer needed to prepare for braces. And the aligners have been refined so much in the last few years that, in the hands of the right specialist, they can be used to treat very complex cases they wouldn't have been an option for before.

Let's dig into some of the new technology that is making patients' treatment—and their life—more comfortable and easier.

WHAT IS INVISALIGN?

The Invisalign system utilizes a series of custom-made aligners that gradually move teeth. The aligners are worn full time and can be removed so you can brush, floss, and eat as you normally would, a big change for those of you who have worn braces in the past!

To fit you for Invisalign, the first step is to scan your teeth and your bite. We send the resulting 3-D images, along with a prescription and treatment plan, to the lab, where they create a simulation of the tooth movements and the attachments, and most importantly, the end result. As a matter of fact, we can perform this simulation during your first consultation and show your expected results. It is amazing technology!

At this point, our expertise comes into play: We adjust the movements, attachments, and the stages of tooth movement, following sound biomechanical principles, according to our desired results and treatment plan. In fact, this is where we spend most of our time in Invisalign cases: modifying the simulation and designing the attachments and staging tooth movement to get a better result. It's fine-tuning, and a critical step in getting the best outcome. We usually go through this process several times, exchanging information with the lab technician, until we are happy with the simulation. Once we finalize the process, the aligners are fabricated and shipped to our office. This process takes about a month, and the patient returns to the office to have them installed.

When we install aligners, we also bond tooth-colored composite shapes called attachments to some teeth in order to help with tooth movement. The attachments are much like a handle on the tooth that we use to create the desired force. As the aligners are placed, they engage these attachments to create the desired vector and amount of force required to move the teeth in the direction we planned.

Invisalign patients generally come for office visits that are spaced anywhere between eight and twelve weeks apart. These visits are necessary for us to monitor the progress of the treatment and make adjustments when needed. We usually do another scan of the patient's mouth at some point during the process to ensure we are moving toward the ideal results as laid out in our plan.

It is important for patients to understand that Invisalign is only a tool; that the results will highly depend on the proficiency of the provider delivering the treatment.

The more consistently you wear your aligners and keep your orthodontic appointments, the better your result will be. At the end of your treatment, the attachments are polished off, and you are fitted for retainers to be worn at night.

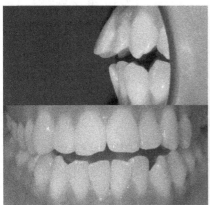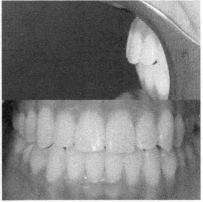

This patient came in for another opinion because she had been told by an orthodontists that she needed extractions and another orthodontist said she needed jaw surgery. These are her before and after photos after non-extraction treatment at our office with Invisalign for 20 months. It is important for patients to understand that Invisalign is only a tool and that the results will highly depend on the proficiency of the provider delivering the treatment.

TWENTY-FIRST-CENTURY BRACES

Braces today are very different than they were in days gone by. There are several different types of braces. I think of them as being a lot like cars in terms of offering various makes and models with differences in performance and quality. For instance, traditional braces require ties over the brackets to hold a wire in place, while self-ligating braces have a door that locks to hold the wire in place.

At our office, we use the highest-end self-ligating bracket on the market, the Damon System. These self-ligating brackets enable us to use mechanics to deliver more constant and natural forces. Generally, we avoid using ties throughout the mouth because they can harbor bacteria and are hard to keep clean. Most of our younger patients love the colored ties, though, and request them, so we still place them on the top front teeth, just for fun. This type of bracket also means you do not need to come in for "reties." All we do is change the colors because they lose their effectiveness after three to four weeks. The self-ligating system retains its effectiveness the whole time, so you visit our office less often during your treatment.

We also use memory wires, the very latest technology in wires. These wires deliver light and constant forces. Our combination of self-ligating brackets and memory wires allows us to treat cases not only more comfortably but with fewer tooth extractions. We absolutely love the results we achieve with them. When you have braces, you usually come to our office every four to ten weeks, depending on what stage of treatment you are in. It is important to understand that braces are not "set it and forget it," meaning orthodontic visits are imperative for treatment to progress and for teeth to move in the right direction.

Don't like the look of braces? For more aesthetic options, there are both clear braces and Invisalign. The clear braces we use are made out of porcelain, so they do not stain, unlike the plastic braces that do stain over time. We offer clear braces on the top teeth, and we avoid them on the bottom teeth because of the chewing forces that that can cause the teeth to wear or the brackets to shatter. Some patients inquire about lingual braces. Both Dr. Giannetti and I worked with lingual braces early in our careers and have opted to no longer offer them, because alternative aesthetic options produce better results. Also, they are very difficult for the patient to keep clean and to adjust to wearing since they sit against the tongue.

The process of installing your braces takes about sixty minutes and is virtually painless. We don't use any sort of anesthetic during the installation process because it's not needed. This appointment is by far the longest one you will have during your treatment process because we like to take our time to make sure that we set things very precisely at this very important visit.

In the first step, our licensed, registered dental assistant will polish your teeth. After that, she will put on a cheek retractor that lets us have a very clear view of your mouth so we can precisely position the brackets. The retractor also helps us keep your teeth dry, which is important because bonding is a very technique-sensitive process and the material adheres much better when the teeth are kept perfectly dry.

After the cheek retractor is on, we apply a tooth conditioner and then a tooth primer. I like to compare it to the two-step process we go through when we wash and condition our hair. In this first step, we use a conditioner that makes the tooth ready to receive the bonding agent. Then we rinse that off and apply what we call a primer to the teeth. These steps assure that there will be an effective bond between the bracket and the tooth.

The next step is installing the brackets. We add composite material to the base of the bracket and the doctor precisely places them on the teeth one by one. After they're in place, we use a special light that cures the composite material so that when it hardens, the brackets stay in place. This bonding process and materials are similar to what your regular dentist would do when you have a composite or tooth-colored restoration.

LETTER FROM A PATIENT...

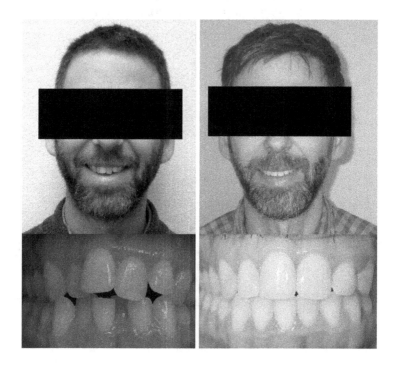

Hi, this is Mitch and I just completed my orthodontic treatment with you. I wanted to write you a quick note to say Thank You and to let you know it was inspiring to be treated by you and the wonderful ladies on your team. I wish I had been able to better know Dr. Giannetti—we shared a wonderful conversation at the end of my treatment, but I only saw her maybe a few times during the course of having my braces.

To provide a brief back story, I have been working on machines virtually all my life, and along the way, I garnered the reputation of being dexterous. Hard to reach assemblies (blind fasteners, etc.) I have generally excelled with. Therefore, as someone who has worked a lot with his hands, when you first put on my braces, I was astonished at your speed and precision. You have clearly reached a high level of mastery, no doubt through many repetitions, but also actively practicing—there's a big difference between going through the motions and actively seeking opportunities for refinement and improvement. Your level of skill can only come from the latter.

The next thing about my experience which was so impressive was your level of professionalism. My observation of this started, again, at the appointment when you put my braces on. During one of your rapid-fire tool exchanges, the pass was fumbled and the instrument hit the floor. Not even slightly fazed, you said "Ohhhh perfect," and kept right on moving without so much as even a slight drop in pace! It would have been very easy (and very understandable) to get flustered in that moment but you stayed perfectly on course.

My observation of this continued with each visit— you (and everyone on your team for that matter) were executing at a high level each and every time I sat down. Consistency like that is very, very hard. As a licensed engineer, I have strived to achieve this, and through no one's fault but my own, it seems I am often one step behind. As in motorsports—one fast lap is relatively easy; a string of fast laps is devastating to your competition.

Once the brackets are on, we select the wire. We mostly start with a very light wire (similar to a piece of floss) that will begin the process of moving the teeth with gentle forces. Once the wires are placed, we will talk with you to go over the special instructions on how to care for your braces, how to keep your teeth clean, and how to floss. Flossing with braces, while more time consuming, is also necessary. We will introduce you to what's called a floss threader, which is a useful tool that helps you to get floss under the wires and in between your teeth. We will also give you samples of different tools to floss with, such as a floss pick designed for braces, so you can choose the one you think you will do better with.

At this point, we'll also review special instructions on what foods you'll have to avoid. Basically, anything crunchy or sticky is off the menu while you have braces, since those foods can loosen your braces or pull the wires off. The good news is that you can still chew gum! We recommend sugar-free chewing gum and, in fact, chewing gum after your appointments helps minimize discomfort.

In about two months, you'll come in again and, usually, get a new wire. As your treatment progresses, we move up on wire sizes until we get to a "detailing wire" that will be used throughout the last few visits to fine-tune the alignment of your teeth and your bite.

You can expect to be seen for appointments every four to ten weeks until it's time to take your braces off. When you come in for appointments, the doctor will evaluate your progress and how your teeth, jaws, and gums are responding to treatment as well. At our office we always take an additional x-ray mid-treatment to evaluate how the roots of the teeth and bones are responding to treatment. We will continue to tailor and individualize your treatment until you arrive at the point where we are all thrilled with the results. Now you understand why we said earlier that braces aren't a "set it and forget it" type of treatment.

When your treatment is complete, we will go over retainer options and schedule an appointment for you to have your braces removed and your retainers delivered.

The treatment time can vary anywhere between twelve and twenty-four months, depending on the complexity of the case and also on other variables such as a patient's compliance and growth.

"BUT DO THEY HURT?"

People who've had braces in the past—and forgot to wear their retainers—are often worried about the pain they remember having after their braces were installed. Thanks to the combination of self-ligating brackets and memory wires with natural forces, the early days of treatment with braces are much, much easier. Most of our patients experience some degree of discomfort because, after all, the mouth is a highly sensitive area and teeth are being moved. You can expect the soft tissues of the mouth to feel slightly irritated with some degree of tooth soreness that typically peaks after twenty-four hours. After the first couple of days, you will likely notice that the discomfort starts to go away as your mouth adjusts to the appliances. I tell patients that their mouth is not going to be hurting all the time. It's more like when you bite down, you notice that your teeth are achy. We will help set you up for success during these first few days by giving you dental wax to protect your gums, and tips on foods that you will want to have around the house as your mouth adjusts.

When I talk about setting up for success, what I like to tell patients and parents is be prepared to deal with a few uncomfortable days. You're not going to want to chew much until you get used to your braces. So for the first two days, you want to have soft foods available. Foods such as smoothies with protein, soup, scrambled eggs, oatmeal, soft vegetables, flaky fish, ground beef, and soft-cooked pasta are some of the options. Once you get past day two or three, your braces will start to feel more normal in your mouth, and you'll be able to go back to most of what you ate before.

One of the best parts of wearing braces has to be the day they come off. At that point, the most common remark patients make is that their teeth feel slimy! Of course, they are *not* slimy, but the braces have become so natural to them that they have forgotten what their gums and teeth felt like without them.

All of this said, it's true that different people have different pain thresholds and varying levels of tolerance for discomfort. Those who experience pain more keenly than most people do may be uncomfortable for longer and take a little longer getting adjusted to them. Sometimes, for instance, the rubbing of the braces initially causes sores in the mouth. We have ways of easing these problems and can adjust the wires to lighter levels of force to reduce the discomfort, or we can give the patient a special mouthwash that is good for soothing irritation. We're happy to move things a little more slowly if that's what it takes to make patients more comfortable.

ORAL HYGIENE ROUTINES CHANGE WHEN YOU'RE IN BRACES

As important as daily, good oral hygiene maintenance is, it takes on even more importance during orthodontic treatment because all the great work being done to give you a beautiful smile can be undermined if poor hygiene damages your teeth.

The most important tools to keep your teeth healthy and your braces clean are your toothbrush and dental floss. Those are the basics. The main change is the way in which you brush, and you will be shown how to properly angle the toothbrush once your braces are on. That's the most important thing, because no matter what kind of toothbrush you're using, if you're not using it correctly, you are not going to be able to clean your teeth properly.

When you come in for your first visit after the placement of your braces, we will evaluate and grade your oral hygiene. If, when you come for your appointment, we can see that you're not doing a great job of keeping your teeth

The most important tools to keep your teeth healthy and your braces clean are your toothbrush and dental floss.

clean, we'll review the instructions on hygiene we gave you so we can see where you need to improve. If the patient is a child, we'll review all these instructions with both the child and the parents, so they can help with the cleaning routine.

Another tool many of our teenage patients like is a floss pick because it's an easier way to floss without having to thread the floss between each tooth. Many patients decide to invest in a WaterPik, and that's a great tool to use when you are wearing appliances as it gets debris out more effectively. If you have an electric toothbrush, keep using it. If you're told that you're just not doing a good enough job of keeping your teeth clean in braces, you might invest in an electric toothbrush, although that's not strictly necessary. Generally, we recommend that you go to your regular dentist for more frequent cleanings while wearing appliances. While twice a year is often enough for most people, if you're struggling with your hygiene, extra cleanings are a smart investment. After all, you want your teeth to look beautiful once they're straightened, and in fact, oral hygiene also contributes in other ways to a good outcome because the cleaner the teeth are kept during treatment, the better the gums respond to treatment, allowing the teeth to move more easily and comfortably. The better the gums and the bone respond, the more predictable the tooth movement is and the better your teeth are going to look at the end.

Several bad things can happen if you don't keep up with your hygiene efforts. The most obvious is gingivitis or gum inflammation, which, of course, can happen to anyone who isn't careful about keeping teeth and gums clean. The big problem that can go along with braces is orthodontic white spot lesions (WSLs). These are white spots that you sometimes see on teeth where the braces were and are caused by plaque buildup. Plaque is bacteria, and those bacteria give off acid as a waste material, which causes decalcification or white spots. So, contrary to popular belief, white spot lesions are not caused by braces but by poor brushing and high sugar intake between meals. White spots are permanent, but they're easy to prevent if you keep your teeth clean and avoid sugary drinks between meals. If we detect them as they're just starting to form, we have prescription toothpaste we give you to prevent the teeth from getting worse, and we enlist the help of your general dentist in helping us avoid them.

REMOVING YOUR BRACES AFTER TREATMENT IS DONE

"Does it hurt to get my braces off? How are you going to take them off?" These are the two questions that often come up as the appointment to remove braces approaches.

When the day comes to get your braces off, we use a special tool that loosens up each bracket to remove the braces. When the brackets have been loosened and the braces removed, we need to clean off the dental glue that was used to bond them to the teeth and is still on the teeth. We have a special polishing bur that is gritty enough to polish the glue off but isn't as hard as the enamel, so it won't damage it. We carefully buff the adhesive off your teeth and go over them with a fine polish so they look just as nice and shiny as they did before. Working with the right tools makes it easy.

Since you need to wear a retainer for as long as you want to keep your teeth straight (for more information on retainers, see chapter five), the next thing we do is take a scan, or impression, for that retainer (or retainers). At your last visit, we deliver your new retainers with instructions, take a last x-ray to check the roots of your teeth and your wisdom teeth, and go over your results. It is very rewarding to look at the before and after photos; patients and parents are always thrilled. It is a great day all around because people are so happy with their new smiles and have grown close to the wonderful team members they've been meeting with through the process.

"DO I GET TO CHOOSE BETWEEN USING INVISALIGN OR GETTING BRACES?"

Some patients come into our office already knowing which treatment they want. At our office, we offer both options, so the patients get to choose whether they want to be treated with braces or Invisalign. Which option you choose has a lot to do with your preferences and your lifestyle. Are you the kind of person who will reliably put the aligner back in the mouth after eating? If not, you might be better off with braces because your aligner won't work if you're not wearing it. Unlike braces, which you don't have to remember to put on, wearing your Invisalign aligner all the time is critical to getting results. We let our patients choose because they know more about their lifestyle and preferences than we do, and we find they're very honest. What has been surprising to us is that children and teenage patients usually do very well with Invisalign, better than adults in fact! That is one of the reasons we love to use Invisalign with teenagers and young children who are going through the first phase of treatment. Adults also love Invisalign due to its aesthetics. We like the fact that the aligners are comfortable and that patients can take them out to brush/floss and to eat the occasional crunchy or sticky treat.

However, the mechanics of braces and Invisalign are very different, and there will always be a small percentage of cases in which we recommend the one we think will work better than the other.

In all cases, we work with our patients to ensure that they are happy with the choice they make and are informed about their options, the pluses and minuses of the modalities, and how important it is that they do their part to contribute to their success.

EMERGENCIES, REPAIRS, AND MOUTH GUARDS

Most problems happen during the first couple of weeks after the braces are installed because the first wire we put in is very thin and flexible, so flexible that it feels like a piece of floss. Sometimes as the patient is chewing, the wire will come out of its little slot. That's a simple fix: we just guide it back into its place. Wire slippage is the most common reason we get a "comfort" call from a patient.

The second most common issue is a bracket coming loose. Typically, this happens because the patients forget the rules on food and bite down on something really hard. Some people chew on a pen or a pencil habitually and forget that's not something they can do in braces. Sometimes the bracket is loosened by eating something like popcorn and hitting a kernel. Occasionally, it's because the patient got hit in the face.

A less common cause for a loose bracket can be something that happened during their installation—for instance, the patient had a hard time holding still, or too much saliva when the adhesive was being applied prevented a strong bond. If this is the case, the bracket will often come off within the first few days after the braces have been put on.

Usually, if something comes loose, patients simply call the office, and we'll schedule the repair as soon as possible so their treatment can progress. We don't see things coming loose very often in our practice, and I think that's partly because our patients are so compliant, thanks to the efforts we make to educate them and set them up to succeed. But if something does break or come loose, we never make our patients feel they've done something "bad." We just get them in as soon as possible and fix it for them. In fact, if a patient comes in for a regular appointment and something is loose, we take care of it during that visit as well. We understand that getting braces means you've got to break some old habits and cultivate new ones, and that can be a big adjustment.

Another common orthodontic problem is a poking wire. This can be due to the fact that teeth have shifted and now there is excess wire in the back part of the mouth, or sometimes the wire shifts to one side, causing it to stick out more on that side. Either way, it can be uncomfortable for the patient as the wire may rub against the cheek when the patient chews or talks. On the day we install the braces, we give our

What's most important for us is that the problem is fixed right away, so that our patients can be comfortable and keep making progress.

patients wax and show them how place it over the trouble area until they get to the office to have the wire taken care of.

And there is no charge for replacing broken brackets or reattaching wires, or any of the common kinds of repair we're called on to make at our office. What's most important for us is that the problem is fixed right away, so our patients can be comfortable and keep making progress.

Another thing that differentiates our office is that we are opened five days per week, which makes it very convenient for our patients to have any issues addressed. If you have an orthodontic problem outside business hours, you will have access to Dr. Giannetti's cell phone or my cell phone to ask questions and get help. On occasion, we come to the office to see patients on a weekend to make sure they are comfortable.

Parents often ask us whether their child should wear a mouth guard when playing sports while they're in braces, and the answer is absolutely yes. We highly encourage it, and we carry special mouth guards they can use over the braces, because even if they already have a guard, it won't fit over the braces and adjust to the teeth as they move.

"WILL I NEED RUBBER BANDS, AND IF SO, WHY?"

It's very likely that if you have braces, you will need rubber bands at some point in your treatment. The time frame in which the rubber bands will need to be worn will depend on how much correction must be achieved. Rubber bands are typically used to guide the teeth into place and help them fit into a better bite. Generally, patients who need a bite correction or who have a bite discrepancy will need to wear rubber bands. Some patients may only need the rubber bands at the very end of treatment, just to fine-tune their bite to make sure it's nice and solid. Other patients will require rubber bands throughout their treatment, while still others may only need them for a month or so, depending on the amount of movement that needs to be achieved.

Rubber bands can also be worn with Invisalign aligners. In fact, we do a lot of bite correction with Invisalign and treat complex cases with it, so we often incorporate the rubber bands into the plan.

"CAN I SPEED UP MY ORTHODONTIC TREATMENT?"

Some of my patients ask if they can speed up their orthodontic treatment. For example, a patient is planning to get married or is preparing to apply for a dream job. In these cases, patients may want to accelerate their treatment. The first and most important factor in keeping treatment moving on time is to commit to coming to all appointments and, in the case of Invisalign, wearing the aligners for the time specified in the treatment plan. Fortunately, beyond that, there are some safe, effective ways to speed up orthodontic treatment.

One option is *low-level laser therapy*. This method uses a very low intensity medical laser to recruit cells that are responsible for moving teeth. It results in faster turnover of bone, which causes healthy acceleration of tooth movement. The application of this laser also decreases pain.

If a patient opts for this method, the procedure is done in the office every couple of months. It takes about twenty minutes and is normally done at the same time as the patient's regular appointment, meaning that there is no need to schedule additional appointments.

Another adjunct we sometimes use, especially with Invisalign, is *high-frequency vibrations.* High-frequency vibrations are effective in controlling pain and, when used with aligners, help the aligners sit against the teeth better, improving the forces delivered to the teeth. In this case, the patient is given a device to use for about five minutes per day at home. An added bonus is that it can also be used any time to control pain. This is especially handy if the patient feels discomfort after a new adjustment, so it can also be used with braces.

Another way to accelerate orthodontic treatment is through the use of *microtrauma.* In this procedure, the orthodontist focuses on areas that are being stubborn. Tiny holes are poked in the gums to recruit cells needed to move teeth. This procedure can be used any time during the course of treatment when the doctor notices that the teeth are not moving as quickly as they should. An example of its effectiveness is that patients who use Invisalign can change their aligners every four days versus every week.[2]

Patients should know that this procedure requires a special appointment that takes about twenty minutes. Anesthesia is given during the appointment to numb the gums. It gets the fastest results but may not be the right choice for everyone because of the use of anesthesia.

When patients indicate that speed is particularly important, we're happy to recommend one of the previously mentioned acceleration options, based on individual needs, as well as tailor their treatment plan accordingly. We can add these options for one additional fee that can be included in the patient's regular payment plan.

Whichever modality you choose, and whatever your treatment plan, we're always here to help you and to cheer you on as you get closer to achieving your goals and getting that beautiful smile you've always wanted.

2   M Alikhani, et al., "Effect of micro-osteoperformations on the rate of tooth movement," *AJO-DO* 144, no. 5, (November 2013): 639–48, https://doi.org/10.1016/j.ajodo.2013.06.017.

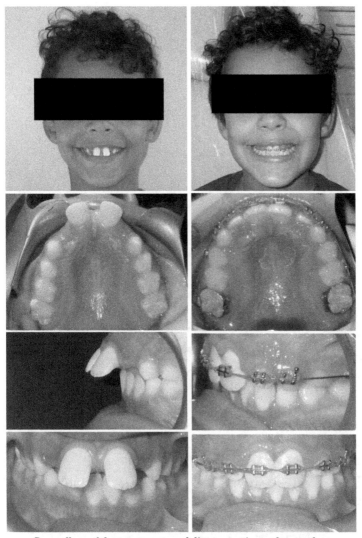

Regardless of the treatment modality our patients choose, they all feel like, at the end, it was worth it. These pictures show a patient undergoing Phase I treatment with partial braces and night-time headgear wear. Treatment was recommended for esthetics and to reduce the proclination of the upper front teeth. When those teeth are proclined, they are more prone to trauma.

CHAPTER FIVE

The Truth about Retainers

by Dr. Booms

Megan had been a model patient. Her case had been a complex one, thanks to severe crowding of her top and bottom teeth. But two years in braces had given her wonderful results and the smile she'd dreamed of. When her braces came off, I fitted her out with retainers for both her top and bottom teeth and sent her home with instructions on how to care for them.

Six months later, she came in with her mom for a retainer check, still flashing that gorgeous new smile. I was really happy to see how great she looked—until I sat her in the chair and looked into her mouth. My heart sank: her bottom teeth had moved and were well on their way to being as crowded and out of alignment as they had been when I first began treating her. I guessed immediately what had caused it. "Megan, you haven't been wearing your retainer?"

Her face fell, and I could see she was near tears. She admitted to me that she'd lost her bottom retainer right after her last visit but hadn't told her parents about it, because she was afraid she'd be in trouble. Her parents didn't know—her smile didn't reveal what was going on with her bottom teeth—and naturally, her parents didn't look into her mouth.

But there was no getting around it, and as unhappy as she was, we had to tell her mom what had happened. Now, we had to put braces back on her bottom teeth and start over—after just six months!

When patients get their braces off, and I fit them for a retainer, their first question is always, "How long do I have to use this?" The answer is, "For as long as you want your teeth to stay where they are." Patients are often unpleasantly surprised to discover how quickly their teeth will migrate back to their original positions when braces come off if they fail to wear their retainers. Unfortunately, biology isn't on your side in this scenario, and understanding why requires a little lesson in tooth movement and how it works.

HOW DO TEETH MOVE?

Teeth are attached to the jawbones by ligaments. During orthodontic treatment, as forces are applied to teeth, the ligaments stretch and compress, causing bone changes that allow tooth movement. Once the teeth are in the desired position, the ligaments are in a stretched state, exerting forces that will pull the teeth back to their original positions unless you wear your retainer. Retainers serve as a template for your teeth, holding them in their final positions as the ligaments restructure around the teeth in their new positions. During the first six months after treatment, the forces exerted by those ligaments are strong enough to shift teeth very quickly if retainers are not worn consistently. As time goes by and the ligaments are stabilized, teeth don't shift as rapidly.

However, teeth *do* shift even after orthodontic treatment and retainer wear. Teeth shift with age just as everything else in our bodies does. Even if you never had braces, the mouth is a dynamic environment where forces created by chewing, tongue pressure, lip and cheek pressure, along with habits such as grinding or clenching, can cause teeth to shift over time. And some situations will cause teeth to shift more significantly than aging and other normal forces does. Losing a tooth, for instance, alters the whole equilibrium of the mouth. All the teeth start shifting toward the space that has been created, and gaps between teeth begin to appear.

Shifting happens more rapidly right after treatment is completed, when your braces first come off. For the first sixth months, the teeth are extremely unstable because the bone and gums need time to readjust to the new position. After a couple of years of retainer wear the teeth will become more stable, but they will still shift, just more slowly than before.

Unfortunately, we see a lot of patients like Megan. They have to come back for retreatment because they either lost or broke their retainer or decided not to wear it anymore. And a lot of adults who'd had braces as teens were told by their orthodontists that once they were done growing, they wouldn't need to wear the retainers anymore. This used to be the common practice.

Even if your teeth have always been straight, the way they're angled in the mouth—slightly forward—means they tend to get pushed further forward over the years. This, along with the bone remodeling changes that happen with aging, contributes to tooth shifting. That's why it's especially common for the bottom front teeth to get crowded as we age. A lot of my patients report seeing this kind of shift. It's more evident, too, because of the way in which our faces age. The upper lip gets longer because we're losing collagen. Young people show mostly top teeth when they smile or speak, but when you're talking with older adults, you'll see more of their bottom teeth.

These more crowded bottom teeth get harder to keep clean and are so much more visible, which can motivate older adults to get orthodontic treatment.

Sometimes a patient will say, "My wisdom teeth are coming in. Will that make my teeth shift?" Not if you're wearing your retainer! Many people believe that wisdom teeth cause teeth to become crowded, but research shows that's just not true. And while there are many reasons a dentist might recommend having your wisdom teeth removed, tooth movement isn't one of them. That said, when you have your wisdom teeth removed, be sure to wear that retainer, because your teeth will shift faster during the healing period following their removal.

LIVING WITH A RETAINER

When you first get your retainer, it may seem unwieldy and uncomfortable, but just as you would with braces, you do get used to wearing it, and most people are comfortable wearing them within a week or so.

Removable retainers come in a couple of different designs. One is a clear plastic, horseshoe-shaped piece that resembles an aligner and goes over the teeth but not the roof of the mouth. It doesn't take up space from the tongue, so it doesn't interfere with speech and is generally very comfortable for most wearers. The other nice thing about it is that it's only worn at night, from day one, which makes it very convenient. Another type is the Hawley retainer, a more traditional design with a metal bar on the front. This covers the roof of the mouth and takes up more space from the tongue, so initially, it does impair the speech more, but it lasts longer than the clear ones and can be adjusted after dental work. It is worn full-time for the first six months, and after that, at night only.

When we finish treatment, we explain the retainer options available, and the advantages and disadvantages of each. But I leave the choice to the patients because there's no right answer to the question of which kind is better except for "the one you or your child will wear." For example, some parents push for the metal one because it's sturdier and longer lasting. But patients who find it uncomfortable—and for people with a strong gag reflex, the design can be a real challenge—probably won't use it. That makes it the wrong choice.

Some people opt for what's called a fixed retainer, which is glued on behind the teeth. It eliminates forgetting to wear it along with the chance that you'll lose it, so those are pluses. This particular retainer works better for the bottom teeth. If it goes on the top teeth, the lower teeth may hit it. It is also a little more challenging to keep clean due to the fact that it's harder to access. You've got to floss under the wire every night, so it takes extra time to keep it clean and the gums healthy. The other issue with a fixed retainer is that it's bonded to the teeth, so if you bite something hard, the retainer may come loose. If it does come loose and you don't get it repaired right away, then the teeth shift. We always make sure that patients understand the limitations and requirements of a fixed retainer, such as not biting into anything hard, and "hard" would include a carrot stick, an apple, or even a piece of baguette. The upside is guaranteed compliance in terms of keeping track of it and wearing it.

CARING FOR YOUR RETAINER

Keeping your retainer clean requires two things most people already have at home: white vinegar and a mild dish soap. Use these along with your toothbrush to gently, thoroughly brush your retainers whenever you remove them to brush your teeth. Try not to let saliva dry on your retainer, because it is the minerals in your saliva that can cause it to stain. You can also use toothpaste as long as it's non-abrasive. An abrasive paste, such as one containing baking soda, can scratch the retainer, which allows it to retain more bacteria and plaque.

WHAT KEEPS PEOPLE FROM WEARING THEIR RETAINERS?

There are many ways people lose their retainers! I've heard stories about parents who had to go dumpster diving when their child left a retainer wrapped in a napkin and it was thrown out either at the school cafeteria or a restaurant. Often, as in Megan's case, a patient will lose or break the retainer and never get around to replacing it. But there are so many ways people can lose or break their retainers that I wanted to share my top five favorites:

1. **My dog ate it.** Yes, really! Dogs and cats just love the smell of retainers. All that saliva and food residue are a powerful draw, plus a plastic retainer is such fun to chew on! Patients who leave their retainers by the bathroom sink or on a bedside table often come home to a chewed up, or at least a badly distorted, retainer.

2. **My grandma put it in the dishwasher.** Poor Grandma! She was only trying to keep things nice and clean, but a retainer loses its shape when it's heated.

3. **I put it in my back pocket and sat on it.** Retainers are sturdy, but not *that* sturdy.

4. **I was surfing and a wave knocked it out of my mouth.** This happens more often than you might think. I always warn my patients not to wear their retainers in the ocean, because a random wave can make it disappear.

5. **I left it on the dashboard and it melted.** Again, heat is not good for a plastic retainer, so a hot dashboard isn't the place to set it down.

But, of course, more often, they're just plain lost, and people get too busy to come back for a new one.

Retainers only work when they're in your mouth, not when they're on

> Retainer use is "nighttime for a lifetime."

your nightstand. As we tell our patients, retainer use is "nighttime for a lifetime."

"HOW LONG WILL MY RETAINER LAST?"

The short answer is that "it depends." The typical life span of a retainer varies. You can expect your retainer to last for several years but not forever. If you're wearing it 24/7, it won't last as long as it will if you wear it only at night. And if you grind or clench your teeth, expect it to wear out more quickly. Imagine having a pair of dress shoes you only wear to dinner parties, versus the shoes you wear to run marathons. You can see that the life spans of those shoes are going to be very different. We usually make a night guard for patients who grind in their sleep, which they'd wear instead of the retainer and which has the advantage of keeping them from wearing their teeth down.

OUR RETAINER REPLACEMENT POLICY MEANS PEACE OF MIND

There's nothing I dislike as much as having to tell patients, or the parents of a patient, that they, or their child, must be retreated because of a lost retainer. After all, the parties involved have put a lot of work into achieving a beautiful result and a substantial investment in orthodontics has been made, so everybody is going to be upset. And we certainly don't want the cost to prevent anyone from replacing a lost retainer, much less put teens in a situation where they're too scared to tell their parents they lost their retainer. But as I've already noted, stuff happens, and retainers can go astray.

That's why we began our five-year warranty program for retainers. When patients get their braces off, they receive two sets of clear retainers and a set of 3-D models of their teeth. If they lose or break their retainers, they can drop those models off at our front desk and come back within seventy-two hours to pick up a new set of retainers made by our in-office technician, at no charge, no questions asked.

When we ask our patients what they appreciate most about our practice, our no-worries, five-year, retainer replacement policy is something they often mention. The peace of mind it gives them is terrific, and that makes us happy too. No more dumpster-diving parents. And if the dog winds up burying your retainer in the backyard, you're covered!

—

CHAPTER SIX

Snoring and Airway

by Dr. Giannetti

D o you snore? Does your child snore? If so, something's wrong and your orthodontist may be able to help you figure out what it is. Don't ignore it, though, because there's nothing cute about sleep apnea, and research shows that the consequences to you or your child's health and development can be devastating.

When my daughter, Isabella, was a baby, she snored and occasionally gasped in her sleep, so it was obvious she couldn't get enough air. I took her to the doctor, who diagnosed her with an obstructive airway. At age two, Isabella had surgery to remove her tonsils and adenoids in an effort to unblock the airway leading from her nose to her throat. She improved for many years, but the symptoms returned. As the years progressed, she began snoring and gasping in her sleep again, and she was constantly sick with a runny nose and watery eyes.

By age ten, she didn't want to participate in sleepovers, because she was embarrassed: classmates made fun of her snoring or said they couldn't sleep next to her because she was so loud. She was sleep deprived, her schoolwork suffered, and she didn't like to participate in activities that required exercise. I took her to the doctor and was given various medications and nasal sprays, none of which seemed to make any difference. As Isabella moved into her teen years, her symptoms got worse, and I dedicated myself to finding a solution.

As luck would have it, as part of my professional continuing education, I registered for a seminar where one of the speakers shared information about sleep apnea, explaining that the adenoids could grow back if they were removed in young children who were persistent mouth breathers. I started putting the pieces together and realized Isabella had an obstruction again.

The adenoids are glands located at the back of the throat behind the soft palate where the nose connects to the throat. When everything is functioning properly, adenoids trap germs coming in through the mouth and nose. A normally functioning nose filters the air and removes germs. However, research has shown that mouth breathing bypasses the natural filter of the nose and makes the adenoids work harder, which enlarges them. When the adenoids are enlarged, they can block the airway. We now know that many children who breathe through their mouth because of significant allergic rhinitis may benefit from myofunctional therapy to help them relearn to breathe though their nose.[3] The central valley of California is the "bread basket of the world," which also makes us the allergy capital of the world! Unfortunately, we see this problem frequently.

One of the best tools to begin evaluating the airway is a three-dimensional radiography called cone beam computed tomography (CBCT), used by most orthodontists. I had the very technology I needed right in my city to figure out whether Isabella's adenoids were

3   Fabiana C.P. Valera et al., "Myofunctional evaluation after surgery for tonsils hypertrophy and its correlation to breathing pattern: A 2-year-follow up," *International Journal of Pediatric Otorhinolaryngology* 70, no. 2 (February 2006): 221–25, https://doi.org/10.1016/j.ijporl.2005.06.005.

causing her trouble. When I looked at her test results, I was astounded to find that she was getting absolutely no air through her nasal passage; she had a 100-percent blockage with 1 mm of measured space for airflow! To visualize this feeling, try taking a small coffee straw, putting it in your mouth and breathing through it. It's impossible and scary. This was not a problem medication could solve. She needed another adenoidectomy.

At age fifteen, she had the surgery, and her life improved instantly and dramatically. It's been two years and she is a different kid. She's almost never sick. She's a straight-A student. She exercises. She's alert and happy. And she's having

> **We were so amazed at the CBCT technology that we now have our own machine in the office and perform this screening on most of our patients.**

the most amazing time experiencing the world through her newly discovered sense of smell. We were so amazed at the CBCT technology that we now have our own machine in the office and perform this screening on most of our patients.

As a parent and an orthodontist, I encourage you to be an advocate for your child's health. Well-meaning, well-trained medical professionals do not know your child the way you do. If you feel something's wrong, trust your instincts. If your child's symptoms don't improve, insist on a new approach.

The classic symptoms of sleep apnea in children include:

- ✓ loud or frequent snoring

- ✓ choking or gasping during sleep

- ✓ night sweats and/or restlessness

- ✓ bedwetting (especially if a child previously stayed dry at night)

- ✓ morning headaches

- ✓ daytime sleepiness or tiredness

- ✓ trouble concentrating

- ✓ behavioral problems, sometimes diagnosed as attention deficit disorder

- ✓ sleepwalking

- ✓ occasionally, tooth grinding

It breaks my heart to think of how long Isabella suffered unnecessarily, and I know she is not the only one. Fortunately, health professionals who keep up with their continuing education are now well versed in the symptoms related to obstructive sleep apnea and can alert you to the possibility that you may need to consult your child's pediatrician or an otolaryngologist (ear, nose, and throat doctor) for a sleep study and a diagnosis. Relatively simple treatment is available for children to enjoy life to the fullest.

SLEEP APNEA'S HEALTH IMPACT ON CHILDREN

Evidence is mounting that sleep apnea's impact on children can have serious long-term effects on their development, growth, and even their intelligence. Studies have shown that children who experience broken sleep can have cognitive, behavioral, and psychosocial problems.[4] They tend to do worse on standardized tests, for instance,

4   Jeffrey S. Durmer and Ronald D. Chervin, "Pediatric Sleep Medicine," *Continuum 13, no. 3* (June 2007): 153–200, https://doi.org/10.1212/01.CON.0000275610.56077.ee.

as well as memory tests and even certain kinds of IQ testing. They often lag behind their peers in school. And unlike adults who are more likely to be drowsy and tired during the day, the lack of sleep in a child can manifest as hyperactivity and acting out, even anger. The diagnosis of apnea is too often missed with these children, who are frequently and mistakenly prescribed powerful ADD/ADHD medications such as Ritalin. Depression and anxiety can also be symptomatic of apnea. Apnea in children is even associated with growth deficiency because frequent waking disrupts hormone production and the secretion of growth hormones.

Of course, if children have a cold or flu, they may snore until it clears up. Seasonal or other allergies can also cause breathing problems that need to be treated. But if the snoring doesn't stop, and given the dangers apnea presents to your child's well-being, you really need to seek help, and sooner rather than later.

SLEEP APNEA IN ADULTS

If you suspect you have sleep apnea, you're not alone. According to the American Sleep Apnea Association, "Sleep disorders, including sleep apnea, have become a significant health issue in the United States. It is estimated that 22 million Americans suffer from sleep apnea, with 80 percent of the cases of moderate and severe obstructive sleep apnea undiagnosed."[5]

And while the most obvious effects—sleepiness during the day, inability to concentrate, and nodding off at the wheel are fairly predictable, a lot of invisible damage to your health is also a consequence of apnea in adults, which is associated with

---

5   American Sleep Apnea Association, "Sleep Apnea Information for Clinicians," https://www. sleepapnea.org/learn/sleep-apnea-information-clinicians.

- ✓ diabetes

- ✓ high blood pressure

- ✓ stroke

- ✓ depression and moodiness

None of these are "minor" side effects, and if you've been ignoring your partner's complaints about your loud snoring or putting off talking to your doctor about your persistent sleepiness or frequent waking, please don't do so any longer. You're compromising your health and safety.

People often assume they don't have apnea because they're not overweight, but obstructive sleep apnea isn't always connected to obesity. Aside from enlarged tonsils, apnea is often linked to a narrow, high, or vaulted, palate. It's also associated with *retrognathia,* which means your lower jaw or your chin is too far back. These are usually genetic in origin, and again, have nothing to do with body weight. In actuality, people with long, skinny necks and chins that are too far back are just as much at risk for sleep apnea as larger people with big, round necks.

Unless they have a bed partner who complains that they snore, many apnea sufferers are not aware they suffer from it. All they know is that they can't sleep more than five hours a night, or they wake up every morning with a headache, or they're fatigued all the time. These are all symptoms of sleep-disordered breathing, which should be addressed by a physician.

HOW IS ADULT APNEA TREATED?

A physician will order a sleep study to determine whether or not you have apnea. Once you're diagnosed, and depending on the underlying cause, there are several modes of treatment.

Typically, adults are prescribed a continuous positive airway pressure (CPAP) machine to use when sleeping. But despite advances in the design of these machines, many people find using them intolerable, and too often, they're abandoned. On a side note, there are some studies that suggest the CPAP intolerance can be related to a tongue thrust or a myofunctional problem and treatment can result in better use of the machine. Unfortunately, many providers are not versed in the benefits of myofunctional therapy and many patients are unaware of the problem. It is hard to believe a misbehaving tongue causes so many issues! In looking for something easier to use, a lot of people will seek an oral appliance, which could be great, but please don't try to buy one ready made out of an airplane catalog! You'll be throwing your money away and doing nothing to help your health, because these are not "one size fits all." It's important to note that these kinds of devices won't work for everyone, and they should be custom-made by a dentist for the best fit. And even when a dentist custom-makes one for you, there can be side effects.

To understand that, it's helpful to visualize that they work by forcing the lower jaw and chin forward during sleep, which increases the size of the airway. The side effect of that pressure is that it can move teeth, which increases the risk of developing a malocclusion and crowding. This is even more likely with an off-the-rack, antisnoring device.

Some adults have surgery to bring the lower jaw forward, which is done by a surgeon in conjunction with an orthodontist. Unlike the appliance, if the surgery works, it has lasting effectiveness. However, it is not a 100-percent cure and does come with risks. But if we see signs of risk in children, we can intervene with fairly minor treatment to potentially prevent problems in adulthood.

Sleep centers are located at many universities, clinics, and hospitals, and there's a lot of good information on the Internet, too, for those who suspect they or their child suffers from apnea. One good site is the American Sleep Apnea Association's website: sleepapnea.org. The Mayo Clinic also has significant resources on the topic on its website: mayoclinic.org. If you suspect you have apnea, nothing can replace a visit to your physician. If you are diagnosed with sleep apnea and you don't want to use a CPAP machine, then seeking an orthodontic solution would be the sensible next step. If your child is having symptoms, you should consult your pediatrician and also your orthodontist because if the problem is a narrow palate, the sooner you can get your child into treatment to expand the palate, the better. Even without a diagnosis of apnea, a narrow palate needs to be treated.

If you suspect you have apnea, nothing can replace a visit to your physician.

HOW DOES PALATE EXPANSION WORK?

To expand a child's palate, a palate expander, which goes across the roof of the mouth, is attached to the top teeth. This device exerts gentle pressure that the parent increases three times per week with a key that opens up the expander a quarter of a millimeter each time. That slow expansion process continues until the palate reaches normal width. The expander then stays in place for another six months while the bone is remodeling and solidifying the expansion. Once that's done, we remove the expander and we're done. A retainer isn't usually needed, because we're moving bone, not teeth. It's very important that this be done between the ages of six and nine because that's when children's palatal features are very soft and pliable and can be treated without pain by this simple procedure. It takes children a little while to get used to it, and their speech will be affected, initially. But children are remarkably adaptable, and within a short time, the whole thing becomes quite routine.

SURGICAL TREATMENT FOR SLEEP APNEA

For adults, the process of correcting the problems that cause apnea is much less simple. Usually, the process has to start with orthodontic treatment. Using braces or Invisalign, we move the teeth to fit within their bone structure, and while patients are in treatment, the surgeon operates on them. The surgeon goes inside the lips and makes cuts in the jaw. It's like breaking the jaw in order to remake it and can be done on either the top or the bottom jaw. Once the jaw is in two pieces, the surgeon moves it, takes the chin portion and brings it forward to advance it, and then puts in a titanium plate to secure it. This, effectively, makes the mandible, or the lower jaw, longer. After healing, I continue to see my patients after the surgery, while they're healing, to make sure their teeth fit together.

This is a major surgery, so I usually tell my patients to expect about six weeks in recovery and a month off work. Those who work from home can take three weeks off work. But in general, they won't want to be out working in a physical space where they have to interact with people or be around people, because their faces will be very swollen. The patient will be on a soft food diet and, obviously, needs to avoid any kind of physical activity that could result in getting hit in the face.

I generally have, at any one time in my practice, at least a dozen people who are undergoing surgical treatment. But because we've learned so much about how to treat children early, I believe we're preventing a lot of future surgeries. If you or your child snores, I hope this chapter will provide the impetus you need to get to your doctor and orthodontist to find out what's causing it. If we're not breathing properly, we're not getting the oxygen our bodies depend on, and the price for that in terms of health is just too high to be ignored.

CHAPTER SEVEN

Do-It-Yourself Orthodontics? Please, Don't!

by Dr. Booms

What would you do in order to save money? It's a fair question and deserves consideration. We all find ways in life to cut a few corners and take real satisfaction in the savings we keep. You might try and fix your own leaky faucet, for instance, and depending on your skills, you could save on plumbing services. If you're really mechanical, you might try to repair your own car, though that can certainly end up costing more than you might have bargained for.

But would you take out your own tonsils? It's supposed to be a pretty straightforward operation, after all, but I've never met anyone who was ready to sign up for that! Yet there are companies out there who are selling do-it-yourself orthodontics (DIYO), and there's nothing simple about straightening teeth. Even people who've managed to get through dental school can sometimes make real messes of people's mouths. I know this because some of those unfortunate patients wind up looking for our help to remedy those mistakes.

EVEN PROFESSIONALS MAKE MISTAKES!

Some people will get DIYO treatment without first having a clear history of their mouth. Issues such as untreated cavities or gum disease can flare up when you start moving teeth around. Other times, a general dentist or orthodontist will move teeth to where they look good, but consequently, the bite becomes so bad that the patient can't chew properly anymore. That means these patients have to pay twice, once to the practitioner who did the original work, and the second time to the doctor who fixed that other practitioner's mistakes. You can see how saving money this way can get awfully expensive!

Some patients will go to their dentist for treatment with Invisalign aligners because their dentist advertises those services and charges less than orthodontists do. What the patients don't know is that often, although not always, their dentist has taken no more than a weekend course in how to use aligners and there's so much more to know than anyone can possibly learn in a weekend. That is why orthodontists go to full-time orthodontic training for an extra two to three years after dental school and continue to have advanced training to update their skills on a yearly basis. Shortcuts in education lead to smiles that may look good but aren't functional for chewing. Very often and not surprisingly, the dentists who did the original work aren't in a hurry to point that out to their patients, and it's not until these patients change providers that the new dentist tells them they've got a problem. That's when good dentists will send their patient to an orthodontist. As one of those trusted orthodontists, I get a lot of referrals from dentists, and I know they'll be checking my work. That is another good reason to see an orthodontist referred by your dentist: the orthodontist's work will have to stand up to your dentist's scrutiny.

Other times, a patient will have substandard work done at a corporate orthodontic practice where the patients don't see the doctor during their appointment, or they see a different orthodontist at every appointment. Even the most well-intentioned orthodontists cannot prevent problems when they are not in charge, and things can go downhill fast. Patients with that experience often show up at our practice for a second opinion.

When even trained professionals can make mistakes of this kind, why would you ever consider doing this work yourself?

THE PERILS OF DIYO

How does DIYO work? You sign up with a company, take some selfies, take your own impression, or go to one of their centers to have your teeth scanned, and a few weeks later, a box containing aligners is delivered to your home. According to those companies, you're on your way to straight teeth.

Sounds pretty simple, right? Well, not so much if you consider the risks you're taking.

In this age of home improvement shows, Pinterest, YouTube videos, and IKEA, most of us can share success stories of DIY projects. The difference is that when I go to IKEA, I buy furniture, take it home, and put it together myself, and the worst that can happen is that the furniture may fall apart. When that happens, it's pretty easy to fix. If not, I can call my handyman and have him come and fix it for me. Even if he says, "Sorry, it's beyond repair. I can't fix it," I can just throw it away, go to the store, and buy a new one—although I'd probably go to a different store and buy it preassembled the second time around. At the end of this little adventure, all this would have cost me is some extra time and more money than I had planned to spend.

But when you sign up for DIYO treatment, no doctor plans your treatment and monitors the progression of your treatment or even makes sure your teeth are in good enough condition to be moved. When patients see me for treatment, first we make sure that their gums and teeth are perfectly healthy. We get clearance from the dentist and communicate our treatment plan with the providing dentist, as we will be a team and in communication throughout orthodontic treatment. If necessary, we can help patients find a dentist, who then becomes part of our team during orthodontic treatment. Only after that do we start moving the teeth according to the treatment plan we tailored to that specific patient. We closely monitor how the teeth are moving and how the body and the gums and the teeth are responding to the treatment we planned.

Things can change during treatment. We base treatment on the average response to it, but the truth is there are different individual responses, which is why we monitor our patients so closely. When the patient comes back every couple of months, we check to make sure that gums are responding as we planned, that the teeth are moving as planned, and that there are no issues. Thus, we individualize treatment based on how each unique body responds. But when you decide to go with DIYO, nobody checks that your gums and your teeth are healthy to start with, and many people will begin without that clean bill of health. I would compare it to having a solid foundation in place before you start to build a house. Orthodontics is the same. If the foundation's not solid and we start moving the teeth, then things can really go downhill: cavities get bigger; gum disease worsens, and teeth start to be lost.

But let's say the patients have gotten that clear bill of health. Even so, once they start the DIY treatment, no licensed professional is monitoring how their teeth are moving.

And a product name is no guarantee. Even if your DIYO aligner is made by a leading, name-brand company, the magic isn't in the product; it's in how well it's engineered for your particular case. While companies such as Invisalign and ClearCorrect make great products, they're really software and 3-D printing companies, not doctors. And while this technology has provided wonderful advances and possibilities in the field of orthodontics, it's a tool, and how well it works depends on whose hands it's in.

If you go to a reliable and skilled practitioner to have aligner treatment, you get so much more than just something out of a box. At our practice, if something is wrong with your treatment or it is not going well, we will work with you and make sure

At our practice, if something is wrong with your treatment or it is not going well, we will work with you and make sure that it gets addressed and that we have a good result at the end.

that it gets addressed and that we have a good result at the end. We're going to work with you and your dentist. But when you do aligner treatment on your own, while your aligners may look the same, nobody's responsible for your results. If you wear this thing as directed, but at the end of treatment, you can't chew properly. Now what? Nobody's responsible but you. And the unfortunate truth is that when you end up at the orthodontist office, you realize that your case is now harder to treat than if you hadn't done anything at all.

People assume that tooth movement with aligners is simple because they look so simple. Aligners apply force to the teeth and cause them to move. When you get them from an orthodontist, those movements are planned with very sound biomechanical principles, taking into account the supporting tissue—bone and gums—as well as the surface that the aligners are pushing against. The software designs attachments and plots the tooth movement, and that is when the orthodontist comes in with expertise to modify the movements to what is desirable and predictable, as well as the attachments. Your teeth have to fit together like a jigsaw puzzle to make sure they will have optimal force when you chew, along with supportive gums and joints. That's all taken into account as we move the teeth.

When you come in to get your aligners, we bond tooth-colored attachments to the teeth to deliver a predictable force system that results in a functional bite. When you do it yourself, you don't get these attachments on your teeth, and an orthodontist doesn't design the force system and movement.

When people choose DIYO, their teeth usually do look aligned. Their friends may say, "Oh, your teeth look great! You paid half the price and they look really nice," but the patients may find that their bite doesn't feel right anymore. If the bite doesn't feel right, it can cause a whole cascade of issues ranging from inability to chew properly to tooth loss. It's just like the IKEA project gone bad: you need to now call an expert to help you fix the problem.

But this isn't inexpensive, easy-to-replace furniture we're talking about; it's your teeth. And now that the damage is done, it's likely to be much more difficult and costly to fix this type of problem than it would have been if you had seen an orthodontist to begin with. Even if your smile looks better, your case is now much more complicated than it needed to be, because you've moved your teeth.

And some people don't even want to spend the money for DIYO aligners. Recently the American Association for Orthodontists aired the case of a patient who lost his two front teeth after attempting DIYO. He had actually tried to move his teeth with rubber bands. Apparently, he'd seen it on YouTube videos. The man gave an interview about all the things he had to go through, all this expensive, extensive dental work, and now he's without his two front teeth. It all ended up costing him $40,000 to $50,000, which is eight times what a typical sound orthodontic treatment would have cost him had he gone to the orthodontist to start with. Not exactly smart economy!

If you're on social media, you may be the target of some of these DIYO companies' ad campaigns, which show beautiful before and after pictures of people who used their service. If you've used your computer to search for an orthodontist, or to research orthodontic treatment, you start getting all these targeted advertisements. They look good, but looks in this case are deceptive and only tell a fraction of the story. What I get to see on my online study clubs are my colleagues sharing all these disaster cases that are now coming to the orthodontists to get fixed.

This market is likely to grow because a lot of the original companies' patents on aligners will expire soon. That and easier access to 3-D printing is why we're seeing more and more clear aligner companies in the market.

COURTESY OF THE AMERICAN ASSOCIATION FOR ORTHODONTISTS, HERE ARE SOME QUESTIONS YOU SHOULD CAREFULLY CONSIDER BEFORE ATTEMPTING DIYO.

If you don't know the answers, you owe it to yourself to find them out.

1. As part of your treatment, are comprehensive diagnostic records like x-rays taken before your treatment?

2. As part of your treatment fee do you receive any in-person visit to a dentist's or orthodontist's office during your treatment?

3. Is only one treatment type offered, such as aligners or a certain appliance?

4. If a dentist or orthodontist is involved with your treatment, do you know the name of the dentist or orthodontist who will be specifically involved with your case? (For example, is it available on the company's website or elsewhere?)

5. How do you know if your teeth and gums are healthy enough for orthodontic treatment?

6. What are the possible risks (financial, health, etc.) associated with your orthodontic treatment?

7. Who can you speak with at the online orthodontic company about your orthodontic treatment?

8. Who is responsible for detecting any issues that may occur during your orthodontic treatment?

9. If an issue arises during your treatment, how will it be handled and who will be responsible for handling it?

10. If a doctor is involved with your orthodontic treatment, how can you contact her or him over the course of your treatment?

11. If an emergency arises, does the company have a dentist or orthodontist in your area that you can see in person?

12. If you are injured or have another dispute involving your treatment, how is it handled—litigation, arbitration, etc.?

13. If you are injured or have a dispute involving your orthodontic treatment, what rights do you have against the person or company involved with your orthodontic treatment?

14. Does the treatment model comply with the dental laws in your state?

Yes, DIYO is cheaper than conventional, doctor-supervised treatment, costing perhaps 60 percent of what it would cost to go see an actual orthodontist. But it's your health we're talking about, not your furniture or car, and the costs in suffering and retreatment can more than outweigh your savings. That's particularly true when a bad bite starts wearing down or fracturing your teeth. Now you've got years, if not a lifetime's worth of restorative work to do just to keep your teeth. Not much of a bargain when you look at that cost.

I've seen patients on social media talking about how "cool" DIYO is as though it's comparable to taking an Uber instead of a cab. This is a very different issue, though, in that you're moving things in your body that are dynamic, and potentially creating irreversible changes. If coolness matters to you, you should know that you can get the latest and best technology at an orthodontic office, which is much better than what you can get with these DIYO companies, and you're definitely going to get a better result.

For now, we are starting to see the unhappy results when treatment like this goes wrong. One DIYO patient put his story on social media. I saw the before and after pictures, and it was very clear to me that his teeth were not proportional, nor was his bite ideal. This patient needed a combination of treatments including not only aligners but also rubber bands, and some teeth needed to be reshaped so the bite would fit right.

Instead, as the teeth aligned, the bottom teeth came forward to match and meet the top teeth. So, when he bit down, he bit on the front teeth only. The back teeth didn't meet at all, which means he couldn't chew with his back teeth anymore. This was a young adult, in his early twenties, who would go on chewing like this. His front teeth would wear down, and as his front teeth grew shorter, he wouldn't be able to make them bigger, because he'd only bite them off again. He deeply regretted DIYO because now he had to seek treatment from an orthodontist to correct all these issues, and it was costing him more.

Another DIYO patient recounted on social media that he noticed his bottom front teeth were loose and discovered his lower front tooth had completely come out of the bone and was slowly being "extracted" by the aligners. A colleague reported seeing a new patient whose teeth were all loose from trying DIYO. It turned out that the patient had active gum disease to start with and as the aligners moved her teeth, the disease progressed, and now all her teeth were loose due to severe bone loss.

Since DIYO is fairly new, orthodontists are just starting to see these cases, and even though I did not see those unfortunate patients, what I do know is that their results were devastating in terms of tooth loss and long-term cost.

We orthodontists are passionate about what we do, and we are very sad to see people suffering because they don't know any better. This is another reason we work so hard to make treatment affordable: we believe high-quality orthodontic treatment should be within everyone's reach.

CHAPTER EIGHT

"How Do I Pay for This?"

by Dr. Booms

S o often, when a new patient has been given a treatment plan, the first question we're asked is "How do I pay for this?" As the mother of young children, I've heard a lot of my children's friends' parents joke when they see their child's first teeth coming in, "Time to start saving for orthodontics!" And in fact, some people do start saving up for treatment when their child is very young, just as they do for college. Fortunately, orthodontic treatment doesn't cost nearly as much as college. You can expect it to cost anywhere from three to ten thousand dollars, depending on the complexity of the case. It all depends where the teeth are to start with and what our goals are.

At our office, we focus on making treatment affordable. We worked with consultants who research American consumers and, in the process, we learned that most Americans have about $500 in their bank account. When we heard that, we realized that the standard model that most orthodontists work with requires that the patient makes a down payment of two to three times that amount, which would exclude most Americans from getting orthodontic treatment in a high-quality orthodontic private office. Clearly, if our down payment is two to three times what most people have in the bank, then most people wouldn't be able to afford treatment, so we had to rethink the terms of payment if we wanted to serve more people. That is why we will start someone's treatment for as little as $250 down!

Why do most orthodontists charge a large down payment? They're looking to cover their initial costs and lab bills, whether that's for wires and brackets, appliances or aligners, and that first appointment is the most costly one from the practitioner's point of view. Orthodontists want to feel secure that they'll get at least enough money down to cover that initial appointment. Some of the big corporate orthodontics companies are aware that many potential customers are afraid of costs, so they'll advertise a low down payment and lower monthly payments, making their care look more affordable. But what a lot of people don't understand is that those payments don't actually include everything they're going to need, and they may be charged for necessary "extras" not included in that original quote—for example, if they break a bracket or miss an appointment, or if their treatment takes longer than anticipated. Also, they may charge extra for retainers, or even for x-rays. At our office, the fee that you're quoted at the initial visit is the fee that you're going to pay, period. And it includes whatever it takes to get the patient the results that we are all happy with.

We don't want the cost of treatment to be a barrier, so even though we may not be the least expensive practice in town, we do work with what our patients can afford in order to make sure they can receive high-quality treatment. For many years, we have been offering low down payments and extended monthly payments, sometimes extending beyond the patient's actual treatment. We don't charge interest in the majority of situations. We work with your insurance company to maximize your benefits, and use a third-party company that specializes in insurance billing and patient billing to make that simpler for you by giving you twenty-four-hour access to your account online. And we have software that will let you review your treatment plan and the various payment options available to you so that you can very easily look at the options and choose a payment that's comfortable for your budget. Once you've decided what works best for you, we take care of the rest.

WE KNOW THINGS CAN CHANGE

Life can throw curveballs, and sometimes during treatment, patients can no longer make the monthly payments they committed to, initially. No problem! We can alter the agreement and extend the payments to reduce the monthly dollar amount. Some patients have a windfall and want to pay a lump sum, and that's fine too. We're very flexible, and we're happy to work with you.

Please don't let costs dictate your choice of a practice!

Please don't let costs dictate your choice of a practice! People who worry about the costs of orthodontics will put treatment off or choose a lower-quality practice because they think it will be cheaper, but the fact is, you can afford top-quality care, and this isn't an area in which you want to bargain-hunt. While the initial estimate may seem less expensive, you don't know what hidden costs will crop up, and lower-quality care very often means a less than ideal result. Yes, orthodontics isn't inexpensive, but if you compare orthodontic services with other dental services, orthodontics is comparatively quite affordable once you take into consideration how it affects the whole mouth and how much work it takes to get a good result. LASIK eye surgery, for instance, requires one appointment and costs you about $4,500. Orthodontic treatment may cost twice as much, but it has an impact on everything to do with your mouth and bite, from functionality to appearance. And if you wear your retainer and take good care of your teeth, that improvement will last a lifetime, whereas my LASIK result only gave me ten years without glasses!

Think of what you pay for your phone per month, or cable services, or your car payment. Now compare the lifetime benefit any of those give you to what having a beautiful smile and a healthy bite offers. Our current average down payment is $750, and the average monthly payment is $130. With that being said we have patients who pay in full, and patients who make a $99 down payment and $99 monthly payment. What is most important is to work with what is comfortable with your budget.

Have you ever chosen a cheaper, lower-quality option because you let price rather than quality dictate your choice and lived to regret it when that cheaper option was revealed to be no bargain at all? I talked at length about the new DIYO in chapter seven, which only exists because people are looking for ways to cut corners on expense. If you're considering this option, please don't! Again, and strictly from the financial point of view, you can run into problems if, at the end of your self-treatment, you're not happy with your bite or other results and have to go through the whole thing again. Suddenly, it's not so inexpensive and, in fact, will surpass the fee that a good private practice would have charged you with guaranteed results. I have seen cases where the patients were so unhappy with the end result that they came to our office for retreatment right after "finishing treatment." Don't let that be you, or your child. You're not going to leave our office saying, "Wow, I paid all this and it wasn't worth it," or "I paid all this money and I'm not happy." The difference is that we stand by our treatment quality and we guarantee our results.

As investments go, the health and attractiveness of your smile is a good place to put your money. Yes, a new car is a lot of fun to drive off the lot, but unfortunately, its value diminishes the minute its tires hit the pavement, whereas if you take care of your teeth, they'll last you a lifetime or close to it. You'll get all the benefits of having a beautiful smile and a working bite throughout your life, but your car will continue to lose its value as time goes by.

If you know that having great looking teeth makes you more employable, more likely to be promoted in a company, and seen as better educated and more intelligent—as multiple studies attest—you can see that the investment you make really does have a dollar value for you or your child that goes far beyond the costs required.[6]

I mentioned college savings earlier. So many of us parents make the effort to put money away for that expense because we know how important it is to our child's financial future to go into the world well prepared. We spend money helping our children reach their highest potential: music lessons, test prep classes, tutors, ballet, sports coaches—the list goes on and on. With the research that supports the positive impact great smiles have on peoples' social opportunities and earning potential, why would you do less when it comes to orthodontics?

6   One such study was recently conducted by Harris Poll for Invisalign. Over two thousand participants were interviewed in March 2016. The study's "Benefits of Straight Teeth" section reports that one in five participants "said their straighter teeth has led to a career upgrade or promotion." "New survey reveals how teeth straightening impacts overall confidence," Invisalign, May 18, 2016, https://www.invisalign.com/news-and-events/2016/invisalign-national-survey-results-released.

And given the negative impact that bullying has on children's self-esteem throughout their life, how do you put a price on preventing children from being teased about their teeth because they're crooked or they stick out? If this is the case for your child, please let the orthodontist know during your consultation. Most of us orthodontists are very passionate about our work, and at our office, we will do whatever it takes to help you provide your child with orthodontic treatment and its positive impact on a young life. In fact, every year we adopt cases that we treat at no charge for such children, who have been prescreened in our Smiles for Kids program.

WAYS TO PAY, AND HOW TO PLAN FOR ORTHODONTIC TREATMENT

Many patients don't realize that they can use their health savings account to pay for orthodontic treatment, and/or a flexible spending account which allows them to use pretax dollars to pay for treatment, saving many people as much as 30 percent. Knowing about this lets patients plan in advance and put money away in those accounts to help pay for treatment. And as I said earlier, we help you maximize your insurance benefits, and take care of the billing for you. In some cases, we've even helped patients find better insurance plans when they've come in ahead of time, so they've been able to sign up for a better orthodontic coverage plan.

Our Growth Guidance program is complimentary and allows for long-term planning. If you bring your young child in for an exam and we determine the child is not ready for treatment, we will see the child every six months or so to monitor growth and development and determine the best time to begin treatment. When we can confidently tell you that your child will need treatment in two years, for instance, that gives you time to plan and prepare for that investment.

Children should not have to live with teeth that cause them social problems or affect their ability to chew. Because we care, we do treat a few patients a year for low or no cost. Every year, the Sacramento District Dental Society holds an event where dentists and specialists screen children who need dental care, and we are among those who participate. Different dentists open up their offices and volunteer their time, and we host an event at our office every year where children who qualify financially get screened for orthodontic and dental treatment. Dr. Giannetti and I generally choose children who have the most severe issues, ones that affect their social life or their ability to chew, and we "adopt" a couple of these children every year from this program to treat them for free. It's a wonderful thing to be a part of, and the families' gratitude for this gift to their children is amazing. Making a powerful, positive difference in someone's life is very rewarding and one of the reasons we're glad to come to work every day.

We strive to support the community that supports us in other ways too: We like to focus our outreach on the community in which we practice because we want to make sure that we're supporting it in return. We regularly make donations to local schools and sports teams since many of our patients are children who go to these schools and play sports and we want to help foster healthy habits in our community.

> **We like to focus our outreach on the community in which we practice because we want to make sure that we're supporting it in return.**

WHY IS ORTHODONTICS COSTLY?

As I mentioned, most orthodontists ask for high down payments because the initial cost of treatment is high, and they're trying to make sure the down payment covers those initial costs, which vary widely and are tied to the quality of materials used, as well as the level of training of the team working with the orthodontist. Like I mentioned before, braces are like cars: there are different brands and there are different levels of quality. We always use the latest technology available, which also includes the most expensive products on the market. We use it not because of its price but because we love the results we can provide and the convenience and comfort it gives our patients. If you are investing in the latest and greatest technology, then your costs are high. We also have an in-house lab that helps us control the quality of our appliances. We used to send everything to outside labs but we weren't happy with the quality of the work we got back or with how long it took to get it back. We've found that having an in-house lab is better because the same person makes all the appliances, and we can give her feedback right away so that she makes things exactly the way we want and the quality is terrific. That means the appliances that we make are very high quality and the braces that we use are high quality too, because in our experience, that helps produce the best possible results.

Different practices focus on different things in terms of investing their money. Our biggest costs are tied to our staff because their expertise and ability is so critical to delivering great treatment. Our staff is very highly trained. Not only have they been to school for registered dental assistant programs but we put them through training specific to orthodontics, and we continually invest in their training so they're up to speed on the newest materials and techniques. Dr. Giannetti and I are part of several study clubs where we get to exchange ideas with colleagues and plan treatments for complex cases. We also attend several continuing education meetings a year, and since we consider ourselves lifelong learners, our average yearly continuing education averages three times that requested by the dental board.

We hold a lot of team meetings, and close the office to do staff meetings and training to make sure we're all consistent with our quality of care. We also have weekly lunch meetings to discuss systems and practices, and our team attends special seminars and meetings several times a year since they play such a key part in delivering the quality of care that we do.

You may be paying for the most spacious and beautiful orthodontist's office in town: if your orthodontist is not investing in training and education, while the office has high-quality furnishings, you may not be getting great quality of care. Which would you rather your orthodontist invest in?

Our commitment is to quality and to making our services available to all who need them. If you've put off seeing an orthodontist because of costs, please call and make an appointment for a free exam and consultation. I predict you'll be pleasantly surprised at just how affordable the best private orthodontic services can be, and we'll work with you to help you fit them into your budget.

CHAPTER NINE

Why Choose Our Practice?

by Dr. Giannetti

Our mission statement begins with what matters most to us: "We are loving, compassionate and respectful of our patients and each other." Even though our patients don't read that mission statement, they feel our commitment to it through how they're treated here: "Your practice is so different! I really feel like you care."

And they're right: we're deeply invested in providing quality care for everyone we treat, and making the experience they have with us as comfortable and welcoming as it can be, from the moment they pick up the phone to book an appointment. None of that is by accident; both Dr. Booms and I have been very deliberate in designing it that way.

FIRST, WE CARE ABOUT YOUR RESULTS ...

... and we do everything we can to be sure they're as close to ideal as it's possible to get, regardless of how much it's going to cost us or inconvenience us. We don't believe in nickeling and diming our patients, and while we're certainly not the cheapest practice in town, we believe that the quality of care and our regard for your comfort and convenience is worth it—and our patients agree.

For example, if you show up with your child at your orthodontist's office for what you think is a simple adjustment appointment but discover, once you're there, that your child has a broken bracket he didn't tell you about, most traditional practices would make you schedule a separate appointment to fix the bracket.

In our practice, we do what it takes to move you forward at every appointment, which is a very different mindset. We always tell our team that "it doesn't really matter what they're scheduled for; we're going to do what it takes to move them forward in their treatment." If patients come into our office for an archwire change, but they have a broken bracket, we're going to fix the bracket first, and then we're going to change that wire.

When parents bring their children in for a "comfort appointment"—because, for instance, a wire broke or something is poking their mouth—we'll use that opportunity to check their progress. If we can see that they're ready to move forward, even if their appointment is still a week away, we'll make the necessary adjustment at that point and save them coming in a second time.

THE DOCTOR IS ALWAYS AVAILABLE

We supply our doctors with special cell phones and give the phone numbers to the patients. That means that my patients have a direct line to me, in the case of an urgent situation, and can text me or call me at any time after-hours, when my staff isn't answering the phone. Colleagues raised their eyebrows at that: "You're crazy! They're going to be calling you for every little thing at all hours." But I've found that people are actually very respectful. I very rarely get called or texted when there isn't a good reason to do so or called or texted after-hours in anything but a real emergency. Some patients have my e-mail and they'll e-mail me whenever they have a question or concern that cannot be answered by my team. Obviously, it's rarely urgent, but I get back to them when I can, usually within a couple of days.

When an urgent situation does come up and patients need treating outside regular business hours, I'm happy to take care of them, even if that means going into the office to see them on a Sunday. That's the level of service that we provide, and I don't think patients are treated in that way at most practices.

In most orthodontic practices, a doctor is present at the office three days a week, and less commonly, only one day a week. At our office, a doctor is

At our office, a doctor is there for you five days a week.

there for you five days a week. Most orthodontist's offices are closed either on Mondays or Fridays. We are only closed if we are at a continuing education course. Having two doctors makes that possible, so between Dr. Booms and me, we can nearly always guarantee that one of us will be available to see patients. And you're in good hands, too, with our clinical assistants, who all have advanced licenses and go through significant continuing education—about forty hours every year—to keep up to speed in their skills. Dr. Booms and I do at least sixty hours per year of further training, too, because there's always more to learn.

WE WANT YOUR TREATMENT TO LAST

As Dr. Booms explains in chapter five, we include a five-year warranty for retainers after we take your braces off. We do this because we know that bad stuff happens to retainers and that if patients lose one, they're all too likely to put off getting it replaced. We don't want that to happen, because waiting means your teeth are going to move back to where they were before treatment. So we've taken away cost and inconvenience, a couple of the big impediments to getting a new retainer when yours is lost or broken.

The replacement retainer is free, and when you get your braces off, we create a 3-D model of your teeth and give it to you. That model, which is virtually indestructible, is used to create your new retainer whenever you need one, for up to five years, and with no questions asked. At most practices, a replacement retainer costs anywhere from $150 to $300, so that's a meaningful saving. If, after that first five years, you want to re-enroll in our retainer replacement program, there's a fee. If you decide that you prefer not to re-enroll, and then lose a retainer, we can replace it for the usual charge.

This is especially good for people with teenagers, or college students, and can bring peace of mind to parents. What we were seeing too often was children losing their retainer and not telling their family about it, because they knew it was expensive to replace. Young people don't want to get in trouble, and perhaps they are hopeful that it will simply turn up, so they just don't mention it. Six months will go by, and mom does a double take: "Why are your teeth getting crooked?" But by the time it's noticeable, the damage is done, and they either have to live with it or bear the cost of retreatment.

Now, with this five-year warranty included, there's no fear, no added expense, and no excuse. I often tell children that "there is no reason for you not to have straight teeth. If your teeth do not stay straight, it's because you've chosen not to wear your retainer, not because you lost it."

THE FEE YOU'RE QUOTED IS THE FEE YOU PAY, PERIOD

In our practice there are no unpleasant surprises in terms of fees, during or at the end of treatment—our fee is all-inclusive. Before you begin treatment, we'll tell you exactly what it's going to cost, and that figure won't change, even in the unlikely event your case turns out to be more challenging than we anticipated. We don't tack on fees, as some practices do.

For example, if we're starting a child in phase 1 (early) treatment, I might recommend braces, and then, at some point during treatment, I realize the child needs an expander, which I hadn't accounted for from the start. Some practices would deal with that by telling the parents, "We've decided we need to do an expander now, and this is how much more it's going to cost." In our practice, we say, "Johnny needs an expander, so let's just get that done next week." We don't charge extra for that, which surprises and delights a lot of parents, whose first very natural response is to ask, "How much more will that cost?" We gave you a fee and we stand by that: no surprises and no add-ons.

We monitor our patients when they've finished phase 1 but aren't ready for phase 2, usually seeing them every six months. We take x-rays as appropriate, take photographs, make sure everything is going well, and let them know when they can expect to begin phase 2, all of which is included in the phase 1 fee. If, during those six months, we discover that we need to do something to prevent a problem from occurring, we make that adjustment—and that's also included in the phase 1 fee. I don't feel comfortable with the whole idea of resetting fees once a patient is in treatment. Dr. Booms and I like to see our patients, get in and do what's right, and get them to the next phase at the fee agreed on at the beginning.

WE'RE A HIGH-TECH PRACTICE

We believe in investing in the very best technology available because it does a better job for our patients, allows us to interact more on a personal level with them, and helps to decrease treatment time. These tools also increase patient comfort level and provide a better experience overall. Yes, these tools are costly. It may sound counterintuitive, but practices using old-school technology are more profitable than those using a lot of new technology. The fact is high-quality technology is expensive and reduces the bottom line. But we feel it's a reflection of who we are as doctors and how we want to practice. Our aim is always to give our patients the best care and the best experience we can, and we couldn't do that nearly as well without high-quality, high-tech tools.

OUR PATIENTS APPRECIATE US AND REWARD US WITH LOYALTY

I always feel that one of the best ways to measure how well we're doing is via patient loyalty. Do our patients enthusiastically recommend us to their friends and family? Yes, they do. In fact, we will often start with the oldest child and then treat their brothers and sisters and then, usually, end up treating the parents as well! It's great to see the children as they grow up and very satisfying when the parents decide to do for themselves what they've already done for their children. Some parents go into treatment along with their child, especially if they have a child who's a little reluctant.

We also have a patient loyalty program in our office that gives discounts for members of the same family because we value that. For example, if we're treating your second child after having treated the first, you'd get a discount. Then, when it comes to your third child, you'd get a bigger discount, and for your fourth child you get a bigger discount because we want to reciprocate that loyalty. Once you're in our practice, we want you to stay. Orthodontics is a large expenditure, and we understand that. We don't want our families to have to make choices about their children in terms of who gets treatment and who doesn't get treatment.

Families tell me, "We can only treat one child right now," which is completely understandable. "So I want you to look at Susie and Donny and tell me which one is worse. Which is the one that we need to take care of first?" We frequently have to help them make that decision. Then, when the first child completes treatment, we move on to the next child and give that discount.

We've always had the philosophy that we would rather spend money keeping our current customers than spend money trying to get new customers.

We've always had the philosophy that we would rather spend money keeping our current customers than spend money trying to get new customers (which is the opposite to the prevailing philosophy of cable TV companies).

Dr. Booms and I are both moms, and I think that gives us a unique perspective on what our young patients and their families need and what they're going through. When I examine a child, I wonder how I would feel if that child were my own, and I go from there. I've been on the mother's side of the chair too. Both of my children have had orthodontic treatment, so I can relate to what the parents experience.

We recognize that everyone has a choice when looking for a practice, and we're honored when people choose us. Very often, we're the third or even fourth orthodontic practice patients have consulted as they shop for the "just-right" practice, and we're almost always their last. What I hear from these people is, "We never got this much information from the other doctors we've seen. We love it here!" That's wonderful to hear. And if we are the first orthodontists the prospective patients have consulted, and they don't seem ready to commit to our practice, I always encourage them to get a second opinion at another practice. I'm pretty confident they'll come back to us because we're a great practice!

WHAT MAKES A GREAT PRACTICE?

In our opinion, a great practice begins with practitioners who listen to *you* every step along the way of your treatment journey because there's nothing more frustrating than feeling unheard. We know; we've been there ourselves.

Great practitioners answer your questions; address your concerns upfront and in an informative, compassionate, and respectful way; treat you or your child with sensitivity and patience; hear you when you describe *your* ideal outcome from treatment; and proceed according to your wishes, rather than aiming for their own idea of what "perfection" looks like.

A great practice doesn't fall back on cookie-cutter solutions to cut corners, because every case is individual and needs a unique treatment plan tailored to the patient's needs.

A great practice respects that your time is valuable and doesn't keep you waiting, and treats you at every visit as a welcome guest, not just an appointment on the books.

A great practice depends on a great team that follows through, exceeds expectations, and creates a great customer experience every time. Creating that kind of experience and building those relationships is something we all strive for every day at our practice. It's our mission.

I can't say enough good things about Dr. Booms. I have four children, each with unique needs that needed addressing with orthodontic care. From the tongue thrust appliance to braces to retainers, the Mara appliance and Invisalign, we have experienced so much. Dr. Booms worked personally and uniquely with their individual mouths and showed her expertise in each situation. Not only is her orthodontic knowledge sensational, but her love and time for each one of my children has been a blessing to all of us.

Jenice Williams

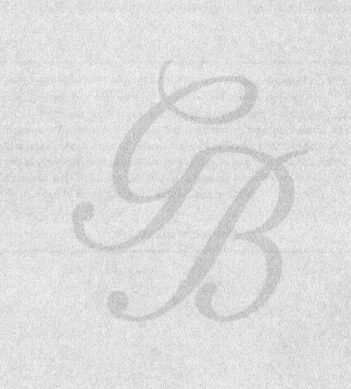

IN CLOSING

If you've been thinking about getting orthodontic treatment but have worried about the costs or the difficulty involved, we hope that you've learned enough from this book to allay your concerns. Today's orthodontic technology is faster, more comfortable, and more precise than it's ever been, so there's never been a better time to get the smile you've always wanted.

Our practice is entirely built on the idea of making it as easy as possible for all our patients to get the results they've dreamed of, and putting that within reach of as many people as possible in a welcoming and supportive environment. We love our patients, and they love our practice, which is why so many of them refer their friends and families to us. We are an owner-operator practice, and that makes a difference in how you're treated here, as well as in the quality of treatment you can expect. We know you have choices, so we strive every day to make our practice the gold standard in our area.

If you've ever wondered what orthodontics can accomplish for you, don't just wonder any more. Call us or visit our website at **sacortho.com** and schedule your free consultation. We look forward to making you smile!

Printed in the USA
CPSIA information can be obtained
at www.ICGtesting.com
JSHW012038140824
68134JS00033B/3128

9 781642 250428